# Teaching IOM: Implications of the IOM Reports for Nursing Education

Anita Finkelman, MSN, RN
and Carole Kenner, DNS, RNC, FAAN

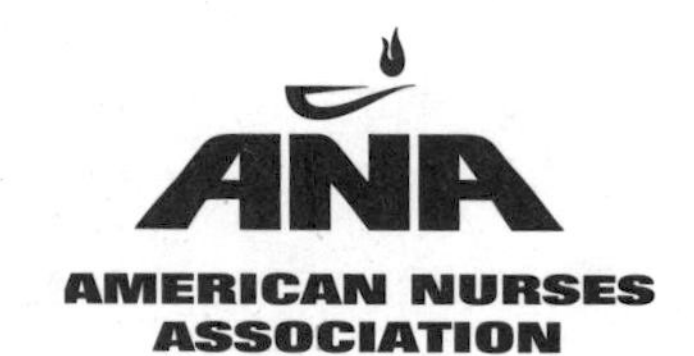


SILVER SPRING, MARYLAND
2007

**Library of Congress Cataloging-in-Publication Data**

Finkelman, Anita Ward.
Teaching IOM : implications of the Institute of Medicine reports for nursing education / Anita Finkelman and Carole Kenner.
p. ; cm.
Includes bibliographical references and index.
ISBN-13: 978-1-55810-240-8 (pbk.)
ISBN-10: 1-55810-240-X (pbk.)
1. Institute of Medicine (U.S.) 2. Nursing—Study and teaching—United States. I. Kenner, Carole. II. American Nurses Association. III. Title. IV. Title: Implications of the Institute of Medicine reports for nursing education. V. Title: Teaching Institute of Medicine.
[DNLM: 1. Institute of Medicine (U.S.) 2. Education, Nursing—methods—United States. 3. Health Care Reform—United States. 4. Professional Competence—United States. 5. Quality Assurance, Health Care—United States. 6. Safety Management—United States. WY 18 F499 2007]

RT71.F46 2007
610.73071'173—dc22 2006100734

ANA is the only full-service professional organization representing the nation's 2.7 million Registered Nurses through its 54 constituent member associations. ANA advances the nursing profession by fostering high standards of nursing practice, promoting the economic and general welfare of nurses in the workplace, projecting a positive and realistic view of nursing, and lobbying the Congress and regulatory agencies on healthcare issues affecting nurses and the public.

Published by
Nursesbooks.org
The Publishing Program of ANA
American Nurses Association
8515 Georgia Avenue, Suite 400
Silver Spring, MD 20910-3492
1-800-274-4ANA
http://www.nursesbooks.org/

*Cover design:*
Laura Hurst, Grammarians, Inc., Alexandria, VA
*Design and composition:*
House of Equations, Inc., Arden, NC
*Editing:*
Steven A. Jent, Denton, TX
*Indexing:*
W. Swanson, Grammarians, Inc., Alexandria, VA



ISBN-13: 978-1-55810-240-8 ISBN-10: 1-55810-240-X SAN: 851-3481

06IOM 2.5M 12/07R
First printing December 2006. Second printing December 2007.

# Contents

## *Part 2 Strategies for Nursing Education*



## *Part 3 Incorporating the Core Competencies in Nursing Education*

## *Part 4 Using IOM Reports in the Classroom*



## *Part 5. References, Readings, Internet Sites, and Other Resources*



## *Appendices*

# Acknowledgments

First we would like to thank our families: Fred, Shoshannah, and Deborah Finkelman and Lester Kenner. Thanks to Elizabeth Karle for assistance with research. Finally, a big thanks to Rosanne O'Connor Roe, Eric Wurzbacher, and Jan Zazada for all their help in preparing this manuscript.

# How Are the IOM Reports Relevant to Nursing Education?

The Institute of Medicine (IOM) series of reports on quality and health care began in 1999 with *To Err Is Human*, which discussed patient safety and errors in health care. Subsequent reports have covered quality of care, leadership, workplace environment, nursing care, diversity, public health, and even health professions education. Health care has responded with improved patient safety, higher quality of care, and reduced errors.

## *Influence of the IOM Reports*

The IOM reports are at the center of the current restructuring of healthcare delivery systems and the movement toward interprofessional work, and they are increasingly influential in funding from research, education, and health policy agencies and professional organizations. They should therefore be at the core of all nursing education programs. Several examples illustrate their impact:

- *Root Cause Analysis*
  The Joint Commission on Accreditation for Healthcare Organizations (JCAHO) requires any accredited organization to conduct a root cause analysis of every sentinel event, defined as an error that results in death or physical or psychological injury. Root cause analysis is designed to uncover the original problem that resulted in an adverse patient event; it includes a critical systems analysis of what went wrong to create the unsafe situation or error. It is based on the premise that most human errors are fostered by system failures, and that finding someone to blame is less useful than assessing how to prevent future failures. JCAHO has developed Root Cause Analyst and Failure Mode Analyst software, and trains users in effective practice, including avoidance of medication errors.

- *Value of Error Prevention*
  Chief Nursing Officer Cathy Rick of the Veteran's Administration (VA) Medical System has stated that one sentinel event costs VA approximately 1.2 million dollars; avoidance of these events thus increases quality of care *and* reduces healthcare costs. The Ohio Board of Nursing (2005) has begun a "Medication Aide Pilot Program" which uses certified medication aides in long-term care facilities to improve safe medication administration, improve quality, and set safety standards including a prescribed curriculum of aide training. Patient information systems and electronic medical record (EMR) systems have proliferated to provide easy and quick access to secured patient information. These systems include medication alerts that highlight drug allergies, incorrect dosages, and potential adverse effects of multiple medications—all designed to safeguard patients.
- *AHRQ Grants*
  The Agency for Healthcare Research and Quality (AHRQ) has issued several requests for proposals aimed at clinical reduction of errors, or policies that promote patient safety and quality of care. In 2005 AHRQ awarded over $22 million in grants that focus on health information technology (HHS/AHRQ 2005). One to Creighton University, for instance, includes use of Personal Digital Assistants (PDAs) to bring drug information to the point of care in order to reduce medication errors.
- *International Efforts*
  The Australian Council for Safety and Quality in Healthcare (http://www.safetyandquality.org/) has applied these IOM reports to safety and quality of care. The World Health Organization (WHO) has entered a partnership agreement with JCAHO to reduce patient errors (http://www.jcipatientsafety.org/show.asp?durki=10858).
- *Research*
  The National Institutes of Health (NIH) roadmap (http://nihroadmap.nih.gov/initiatives.asp) for research initiatives includes interprofessional or interdisciplinary research, strongly recommended in the IOM reports. It calls for "Training for a New Interdisciplinary Research Workforce" and a "Second Phase of the NIH Roadmap Exploratory Centers for Interdisciplinary Research." NIH has called for planning grants for the translation of science to clinical practice, recognizing the need to move science from the bench to the point of care where it can change patient outcomes. The Robert Wood Johnson Foundation has invited proposals for an interdisciplinary nursing quality research initiative to "generate, disseminate and translate research to improve quality of care."
- *Nursing Shortage*
  The proposed Nursing School Capacity Act of 2005 (HR 2184)—still in committee at press time—would authorize a study by the IOM to examine the regulatory, educational, salary, and workplace characteristics that have led to the nursing shortage. This legislation is linked to the IOM's previous work *Nursing*

*Focus: Keeping Patients Safe: Transforming the Work Environment for Nurses* (2004), which suggested that the current nursing shortage is a significant patient safety issue. This report also shows that nurses are the glue that holds healthcare organizations together at the point of care. They serve as integrators to determine patient needs and to alert other professionals who are not at the bedside or in the community clinics. If a nurse does not provide the surveillance function for the healthcare team, significant patient data are lost, and often physicians and other professionals are not alerted to an impending problem. But, as *Transforming* demonstrates, we cannot continue to provide nursing care the way we always have. Some of the work needs to be delegated to others, and some needs to be transformed by the use of technology.

- *Advanced Education*
  The American Association of Colleges of Nursing (AACN) advocates a Doctor of Nursing Practice (DNP) program to keep highly educated nurses at the point of care and to apply evidence-based practice and research to patient outcomes and quality of care. AACN also backs Clinical Nurse Leader (CNL) education in recognition of the integrator role, to coordinate services for patients and their families at the point of care.
- *Geriatric Care*
  The Bureau of Health Professions (BHP) currently has calls out for building capacity in geriatric education (HRSA-06-012), recognizing that the world's population is aging and that to provide quality care we need nurses educated in their special needs. IOM recognized the importance of care for the elderly and the chronically ill when it set the Priority Areas of Care.
- *Workforce Diversity*
  Grants are aimed at increasing the mix of ethnic groups among nurses so that they can provide more culturally sensitive, appropriate care. The grant application for Primary Care Services Resource Coordination and Development focuses on the need for an integration of services to decrease fragmentation of care by specialists, some of which is caused by inadequate consideration of diversity in patient populations, and to increase quality of care.
- *Simulation Tools*
  Funding for simulation centers to promote interdisciplinary education has increased over the past five years. The Voluntary Hospital Association Health Foundation has funded projects that support best practices and health outcomes through simulation. The Center for Medical Education and Innovation at Riverside Methodist Hospital in Columbus, Ohio is one such project. The Bureau of Health Professions Education, Centers for Disease Control and Prevention (CDC), and other governmental agencies have sponsored such projects to deal with bioterrorism and the need for a coordinated interdisciplinary response to natural disasters such as hurricanes, earthquakes, and tsunamis. These simulation labs include Uniform Health Services University, Washington, DC; University of Maryland College of Nursing, Baltimore, MD; University of

Illinois at Chicago Colleges of Public Health, Pharmacy, Medicine, and Nursing; University of Oklahoma Health Sciences Center College of Public Health-Bioterrorism; and Colleges of Nursing, Medicine, Pharmacy, and Allied Health for interdisciplinary simulation training, University of Wisconsin Madison.

## *Implications for Nursing Education*

Clearly there is great movement in healthcare organizations (HCOs) and in government to make changes and improve. It is not enough to reform just healthcare delivery systems; we need safety and quality strategies to resolve problems in clinical settings, and strategies for government and local communities. The report on health professions education identifies the core competences for health professions, but nurse educators would be wrong to ignore the other reports as irrelevant to education. A barrier between practice and education may undermine care, jeopardize safety, and leave nursing behind other health professions that recognize the importance of all the IOM reports and use them to guide decisions about curriculum and clinical learning experiences. New graduates who enter the job market not prepared for the new quality improvement environment will require additional costly orientation and training. Their frustration at being left behind their peers will increase attrition, and with the nursing shortage, retention of new graduates is critical.

Students need to understand and apply the IOM reports. This means that faculty must be familiar with the content and incorporate it into curricula and clinical nursing experiences. Consider the following questions and their impact on nursing education, curricula, and clinical application:

- What is the safety problem?
- What types of errors occur?
- What methods are used to analyze errors to prevent further errors?
- How does a nurse affect patient safety?
- Does the educational environment support a blame-free culture when errors are made?
- What are HCOs, government, insurers, and professional organizations doing to improve care? Is it effective?
- What is quality care?
- How is quality care assessed? What is the status? What needs improvement?
- What are the six improvement aims and how do they apply to nursing practice?
- Do students recognize the importance of self-evaluation, near misses, and surveillance in their practice?
- How does a nurse affect quality care?
- What is the framework for the National Healthcare Quality Report? Where can a nurse access the annual report? Why would these data be important? How

might these data be used in nursing research to improve nursing curricula and clinical experiences?

- What role does leadership play in improving care? How does this relate to nursing as a profession and to an individual nurse? How do we prepare students to be leaders?
- What are the critical issues in the report on workplace environment and nursing care? How might this information be used to improve nursing care? What are the implications for nursing education?
- What has the nursing profession done to improve care, such as ANA, specialty organizations, and so forth?
- Are students able to meet the core health professions education competencies: patient-centered care, interdisciplinary teams, evidence-based practice, quality improvement, and informatics?
- What changes have been made to increase interprofessional educational experiences?
- What is the concern about diversity in health care? How might this be changed? What impact does it have on a nurse and practice?
- What are the priority areas of care? How might they be incorporated into curricula? How are they used in assessing and improving care?
- What are the major issues related to public health? Why is this important? How does Healthy People serve as a critical resource?
- What is the role of evidence-based practice? How can we continually improve and expand nursing research?
- Why is understanding of the change process important?
- How much content and experience related to informatics and medical technology are included in curricula?
- How can we increase teamwork and team experiences?

## *Safety and Quality Care*

The ANA position statement on safety and quality states that the "future direction and focus of practice of nursing, as well as the articulation of nursing's unique contributions to consumers and health policy makers, depends on clearly measuring nursing's impact on patient safety and quality of care" (ANA, 2004). In 1998, the ANA House of Delegates approved an action report, *Shared Accountability in Today's Work Environment.* Prepared before the landmark 1999 IOM report on patient safety, it emphasized four strategies:

- Educate policy-makers and the public on the effects of downsizing, restructuring, and reorganizing that lead to breakdowns in safety and quality.
- Work with other healthcare organizations to identify and correct systems errors that lead to patient injuries.

- Support the role of the professional nurse in correcting systems errors through quality improvement initiatives and protect the nurse by enacting whistle-blower legislation.
- Educate regulators and accrediting bodies on the dangers of the criminalization of healthcare errors.

These strategies, which also appear in IOM (1999) and other national reports, demonstrate that the nursing profession is committed to safety.

The ANA action report considered practice and healthcare delivery; another critical factor can have a long-term effect on safety, namely what nursing students are learning about patient safety and quality. Maddox, Wakefield, & Bull (2001) discuss the need for changing educational experiences. They pose several questions for the nursing profession:

- Do nurses and other members of the healthcare delivery team have the same expectations for individual performance in the interdisciplinary healthcare team?
- Do nurse educators have the working knowledge and experience of technical and human factors (including organizational) required in setting new expectations and in facilitating learning experiences for interdisciplinary teams? Nurse educators need to understand cultural differences in patient populations and the workforce, cultural factors such as the structure of the organization, the significance of the institution's mission and core values on the enterprise, financing of health care, and billing, coding, and reimbursement issues, to name a few areas of knowledge. Other technical issues include patient information systems, monitoring equipment, new hospital equipment and safety issues in its use, and the relation of the Health Information Portability and Accountability Act (HIPAA) to patient information and access to medical records.
- Do we teach and model effective relationship management and communication skills when facing power gradients? (Power gradients are differences in status and influence between health professionals—mainly between nurses and physicians. In many instances power or perceived power of an individual is related to status, educational level, and financial impact on the organization as well as the legitimate or perceived authority of the individual.)

These questions suggest new research to increase nursing's understanding of patient safety and its relationship to nursing care and the role of nurses. They are part of the rationale for the new nursing role of CNL as recommended by AACN in its white paper (2003), which emphasizes leadership, care coordination, financial management, and knowledge of information systems, as well as increasing bachelor's level education in delegation, leadership, informatics, finance, and organizational structure and its impact on healthcare outcomes.

ANA and the American Academy of Nursing (AAN) have both been involved in "Quality" work. They have provided nursing representation to the National Quality Forum. ANA has taken the lead in developing quality indicators used in Nursing's Report Card for benchmarking healthcare delivery systems' quality of care.

Despite this endorsement of the IOM reports by ANA, AAN, the National Institute of Nursing Research (NINR), and AHRQ, many health professionals question the need for IOM information to be included in curricula. But it is changing every aspect of healthcare delivery and patient care. The business of our educational institutions is to produce graduates capable of rendering safe, quality care. And with funding streams so short, educational institutions are driven to diversify financial resources through service learning, educational programs, and research grants. Given the mounting evidence that IOM findings are driving funding, we should be more aware of these reports and teach our students why they are important. The authors of this text realize that in order to achieve that goal, information must be presented in a concise, usable fashion. To that end, this book presents strategies for integrating the IOM material into the curriculum. This integration at the point of education is the core purpose of this text, which is structured as summarized below:

- Part 1 sets the context for the book with an overview of the critical IOM reports. (Eight of the appendices list the recommendations of the major reports.)
- Part 2 examines nursing's general educational strategic responses and issues.
- Part 3 presents specific strategies for integrating safety and quality into nursing education, framed on the five core competencies named in the 2003 report, *Health Professions Education.*
- Part 4 presents a variety of tools that may be used to further guide students as they learn about the IOM reports and how to apply this information to their practice.
- Part 5 lists the references used throughout Parts 1 through 4, supplemented with recommendations for further reading.
- In addition to the recommendations of several of the key reports, the appendices include a discussion of Suzanne Gordon's *Nursing Against the Odds*, a critical portrait of modern nursing.

# Part 1

# Report Summaries and Recommendations

The IOM reports began with President Bill Clinton's Advisory Commission on Consumer Protection and Quality in the Healthcare Industry, established as a short-term commission in 1997. The purpose of the commission was to advise President Clinton about the impact of healthcare delivery system changes on quality, consumer protection, and the availability of needed services (Wakefield, 1997). It investigated many aspects of quality care and the changes needed to improve care.

In 1999 the commission released its final report, *Quality First: Better Healthcare for all Americans*. Appendix A lists the commission's recommendations. This effort led IOM to begin the Quality of Healthcare in America project in 1998. The purpose of this initiative is to respond to issues identified in the Presidential Commission's report with strategies to improve healthcare quality over the next 10 years. It has produced IOM reports on these topics:

- Safety:
  *To Err Is Human* (1999)
  *Patient Safety: Achieving a New Standard of Care* (2004)
- Quality:
  *Crossing the Quality Chasm* (2001)
  *Envisioning the National Healthcare Quality* (2001)
  *Priority Areas for National Action: Transforming Healthcare Quality* (2003)
- Leadership:
  *Leadership By Example: Coordinating Government Roles in Improving Healthcare Quality* (2003)
- Public Health:
  *The Future of the Public's Health in the 21st Century* (2003)
  *Who Will Keep the Public Healthy?* (2003)
  *Unequal Treatment: Confronting Racial and Ethnic Disparities in Healthcare* (2002)
  *Guidance for the National Healthcare Disparities Report* (2002)

- Nursing:
  *Keeping Patients Safe: Transforming the Work Environment for Nurses* (2004)
- Health Professions Education:
  *Health Professions Education: A Bridge to Quality* (2003)

These reports are available on the Internet at the sites listed in the Reference section.

## *Safety Reports*

### To Err Is Human (1999)

### Patient Safety: Achieving a New Standard for Care (2004b)

*To Err Is Human* (IOM, 1999) describes the current national patient safety problem; it has had a significant impact on the public's view of health care. *Patient Safety* (IOM, 2004b) discusses in more detail one recommended strategy for improving patient safety, defined "as freedom from accidental injury." Patient safety improvement will require major changes in safety and quality of care. Multiple stakeholders must commit to these changes, including a revamping of patient information systems.

Ensuring patient safety requires a comprehensive approach, and we cannot rely on a single solution. The 1999 report emphasizes that the workplace must not simply punish individuals for errors. Instead, root cause analysis must be conducted to determine individual practice and system problems that result in errors. This means a standardized method of solving problems. The expectation is that healthcare organizations will then use these data to eliminate or at least reduce the system problems that compromise patient safety. Safe care does not imply that the care is then of higher quality; however, safe care does increase the likelihood of quality care. It would be easy to say that a strong regulatory and enforcement approach is the strategy for solving this problem. But use of appropriate technology is another means to reduce errors. A national mandatory reporting system for errors will also provide useful information to improve safety. Finally, in any of the recommended strategies, leadership is critical.

Next to recognition of the high level of errors, the most important conclusion from the report is the need to change to a nonpunitive, blame-free environment. If a survey asked healthcare providers what is the most common type of error, the prevailing response would probably be that individual providers make errors. Providers would also point out that they are at risk if they report errors. This is a simplistic view of errors, and avoids addressing the more significant effect of systems and processes on errors. "Building safety into processes of care is a more effective way to reduce errors than blaming individuals" (IOM, 1999, p. 4). It is much simpler to blame an individual, and this punitive approach has been a tradition in healthcare organizations. It has left us with an environment of fear where individual staff members are reluctant to report errors or near misses. It ignores the critical fact that errors also provide important information about how the system is working, and this information can be used to improve care. Latent or unnoticed errors are the most problematic: they can later lead to more complex errors. It is, however, much easier to address active errors, which are more visible, and miss the latent errors or errors removed from the control of the direct care staff such as equipment problems, environmental issues, and management decisions.

*To Err Is Human* concludes by identifying five critical principles in the design of safe healthcare systems: (1) provide leadership, (2) respect human limits in process design, (3) promote effective team functioning, (4) anticipate the unexpected, and (5) create a learning environment. All the recommendations from the report are described in Appendix B.

*Patient Safety: Achieving a New Standard for Care* (IOM, 2004b) continues the exploration of safety issues and recommendations found in *To Err Is Human.* In the process of care healthcare providers need to: (1) access complete patient information, (2) understand the implications of environmental factors such as waiting time to receive care, bed availability, and so on, (3) use information about infectious diseases to decrease patient risk, and (4) appreciate the implications of chronic illness and how these may affect care needs. Each of these elements depends on accurate, timely, and accessible information in the form of a comprehensive electronic health record (EHR). The EHR will help to implement best practice and evidence-based care and facilitate standardization.

## *Quality Care Reports*

### Crossing the Quality Chasm (2001)

### Envisioning the National Healthcare Quality Report (2001)

### Priority Areas for National Action: Transforming Healthcare Quality (2003)

These three reports consider a new health system for the twenty-first century. According to *Crossing the Quality Chasm* (IOM, 2001a), the nation's healthcare delivery system requires fundamental change. At the same time the system has experienced rapid change due to new medical science, new technology, rapid availability of information, and other factors. The system is fragmented and poorly organized, and does not use its resources efficiently. This report identifies quality as a system property with six important improvement aims. Health care should be (1) safe, (2) effective, (3) patient-centered, (4) timely, (5) efficient, and (6) equitable. All healthcare constituents or stakeholders, including policy-makers, purchasers, regulators, health professionals, healthcare trustees and management, and consumers must commit to a national agenda of the six aims for improvement. The goal is to raise the quality of care to unprecedented levels. (The recommendations from this report are included in Appendix C.) In addition, the report states 10 rules to guide major stakeholders through collaboration to reach positive outcomes. These rules are drawn from the work of Donald Berwick

**TABLE 1-1 Guidelines to Stakeholders for Collaborative Healthcare Reform: Status Quo Compared to Berwick 2003**

| *Current Approach* | *New Rule* |
|---|---|
| Care is based primarily on visits. | Care is based on continuous healing relationships. |
| Professional autonomy drives variability. | Care is customized according to patient needs and values. |
| Professionals control care. | The patient is the source of control. |
| Information is a record. | Knowledge is shared and information flows freely. |
| Decision-making is based on training and experience. | Decision-making is evidence-based. |
| *Do no harm* is an individual responsibility. | Safety is a system priority. |
| Secrecy is necessary. | Transparency is necessary. |
| The system reacts to needs. | Needs are anticipated. |
| Cost reduction is sought. | Waste is continuously decreased. |
| Preference is given to professional roles over the system. | Cooperation among clinicians is a priority. |

*Source:* Berwick, 2003.

(2003). He also notes the fundamental differences between his new rules and the current system. These differences are summarized in Table 1-1.

*Envisioning the National Healthcare Quality Report* (IOM, 2001b) takes the process a step further with a framework for collecting annual data about healthcare quality, which will reveal the quality of the nation's healthcare delivery system. This analysis will be compiled annually by AHRQ. "The National Healthcare Quality Report should serve as a yardstick or the barometer by which to gauge progress in improving the performance of the health care delivery system in consistently providing high-quality care" (IOM, 2001b, p. 2). The focus of the report is not public health but rather how the healthcare delivery system performs in providing personal health care. In addition, the report discusses healthcare from a broader perspective than the performance of individual providers such as hospitals. The report should not duplicate quality report cards that many individual healthcare organizations currently use to measure their own performance. The quality report should assist policy-makers and should also be accessible and relevant to consumers, purchasers, providers, educators, and researchers.

The design of the annual quality report builds on the definition of quality used in the various IOM reports. Quality is "the degree to which health services for individuals and populations increase the likelihood of desired health outcomes and are consistent with current professional knowledge" (IOM, 1990, p. 21). The quality report follows the most common approach to quality care assessment, derived from Donabedian's (1996, 1980) three elements of quality: structure, process, and outcomes. It is clear that health quality does not mean that all desired outcomes will necessarily be reached, and that a patient who receives care below the quality standard may still reach the desired outcomes. In addition, the approach selected for the report recognizes the influence of the patient: what outcome the patient wants, how the patient's preferences influence treatment, and consumerism. Appendix D shows a matrix of the two dimensions of the quality report framework. The annual national healthcare quality report can be accessed at the AHRQ site at http://www.ahrq.gov/qual/nhqr03/nhqrsum03.htm.

*Priority Areas for National Action* (IOM, 2003a) begins by recognizing that every aspect of care cannot be assessed annually, nor would this approach offer any advantage. The increase of chronic conditions in the United States has had a major impact on the system and is an important factor in identifying the priority areas. More people are living longer and with chronic illnesses, mostly because of advances in medical science and technology. Many of these patients also have comorbid conditions; this increases the complexity of their problems and requires more collaborative health care. The Department of Health and Human Services (DHHS) uses three criteria to set priorities: (1) impact or extent of burden, (2) improvability or extent of the gap between current practice and evidence-based practice, and (3) inclusiveness or the relevance of an area to a broad range of individuals. The priorities are discussed in more detail in Part 2.

*Priority Areas* adds another building block to the national initiative to improve the quality and safety of healthcare. Earlier reports identify serious quality and safety concerns in health care delivery. But every part of care cannot be evaluated. The report specifies the 19 priority areas to begin with. Over time the priority areas will change as new needs arise and outcomes in priority areas improve; however, the annual report's framework should not change greatly unless it proves to be inadequate.

## *Leadership Report*

### Leadership by Example: Coordinating Government Roles in Improving Healthcare Quality (2003)

This report explores the characteristics of an infrastructure that will foster quality. Six government programs—Medicare, Medicaid, State Children's Health Insurance Program (SCHIP), the Department of Defense (DOD) TRICARE and TRICARE for Life programs, the Veterans Health Administration (VHA), and the Indian Health Services (IHS) program—are examined for quality enhancement processes (IOM, 2003b). These six programs serve about a third of all Americans. The difficulty with implementation of the recommendations in the IOM reports has been the lack of reliable, valid indicators of quality. This report stresses the need for the U.S. government to lead in establishing quality performance measures and improving safety and quality of care.

The federal government serves in four roles in healthcare delivery, which makes it uniquely suited to move the quality initiative forward. It serves as *regulator* when it sets minimum acceptable performance standards. It is the largest *purchaser* of care through six major government health programs, and thus can have a major impact on other purchasers of care. As a *provider* of care for veterans, military personnel and their dependents, and Native Americans, the federal government can implement model quality improvement programs and gather data about their outcomes, programs that could then be used by other providers. Finally, it is a *research sponsor*, particularly in applied health services research. The report's recommendations are found in Appendix E.

## *Public Health Reports*

### The Future of the Public's Health in the 21st (2003)

### Who Will Keep the Public Healthy? (2003)

### Unequal Treatment: Confronting Racial and Ethnic Disparities in Healthcare (2002)

### Guidance for the National Healthcare Disparities Report (2002)

Two of these reports—*The Future of the Public's Health in the Twenty-first Century* (IOM, 2003c) and *Who Will Keep the Public Healthy?* (IOM, 2003d)—deal with public health. *Unequal Treatment: Confronting Racial and Ethnic Disparities in Healthcare* (IOM, 2002a) and *Guidance for the National Healthcare Disparities Report* (IOM, 2002b) are concerned with disparities in health care. The public health reports discuss the problems in the system and offer recommendations for improvement. Part of the current atmosphere of change is the need to instill a vision of public health, which has been identified as *healthy people in healthy communities* (*Healthy People 2010*). This vision of the future of public health recognizes that "health is a primary good because many aspects of human potential such as employment, social relationships, and political participation are contingent on it" (IOM, 2003c, p. 2). Public health affects citizens in their lifestyle, income, work status, mortality and morbidity, education, and family life. But public health has frequently been overlooked in the broad view of the nation's health. The key points of the action plan in *The Future of the Public's Health,* found in Appendix F, include a population health approach, public health systems, infrastructure, partnerships, accountability, evidence, and communication.

*Who Will Keep the Public Healthy?* (IOM, 2003d) addresses public health needs in a world affected by globalization, rapid travel, scientific and technological advances, and demographic changes. Effective response to public health problems requires well-prepared professionals. "A public health professional is a person educated in public health or a related discipline who is employed to improve health through a population focus" (IOM, 2003d, p. 4). This report explores the educational needs required to improve public health; its recommendations are found in Appendix G.

The other two reports, *Unequal Treatment: Confronting Racial and Ethnic Disparities in Healthcare* (IOM, 2002a) and *Guidance for the National Healthcare Disparities Report* (IOM, 2002b) focus on disparities in health care and their impact on the nation's public health. They identify major concerns about racial, ethnic, geographic, and socioeconomic inequities. Healthcare disparities occur consistently across a variety of illnesses and delivery services. They are associated not with specific types of illnesses but a broad spectrum.

The findings of the Sullivan Commission (2004), though not one of the IOM reports, are relevant. It examines disparities in health care and concludes that a key contributor to this growing problem is the disparity of the nation's health professional workforce. This imbalance impedes minorities' access to health care as well as understanding of their needs. The commission suggests that the solution is to increase the number of minority health professionals. This translates into increased admittance into professional schools, something that the United States has historically failed to accomplish; today, with increased competition for positions in nursing, this problem can only grow. Even when minority students are admitted they do not always graduate.

The American Indian Success Program at the University of Oklahoma Health Sciences Center College of Nursing is cited by the Sullivan Commission as a model program in meeting the needs of Native Americans. This project, funded by the IHS, is dedicated to the recruitment, retention, and graduation of eligible Native American nursing students from the baccalaureate program. The overall goal is to prepare Native American nurses to provide healthcare services to the state's Native American citizens. Critical elements of this program include academic counseling, resource referral, and scholarships. This program dovetails with the Human Resources and Services Administration (HRSA) grant for Cultural Diversity and Training, which includes leadership development. The object of such programs is to help minority students to enter nursing with the ultimate goal of culturally sensitive, high-quality care for minority patients and their families.

*Guidance for the National Healthcare Disparities Report* (IOM, 2002b) outlines the annual National Healthcare Disparity Report, which is available on the Internet at http://www.ahrq.gov/qual/nhdr03/nhdrsum03.htm. This report tracks four measurements: (1) socioeconomic status, (2) access to the healthcare system, (3) healthcare services and quality, and (4) geographic disparities in health care.

## *Nursing Report*

### Keeping Patients Safe: Transforming the Work Environment for Nurses (2004)

*Keeping Patients Safe: Transforming the Work Environment of Nurses* (IOM, 2004a), although germane to nursing in any setting, focuses on acute care. It addresses critical quality and safety issues with an emphasis on nursing care and nurses, particularly the work environment. As the report states, "When we are hospitalized, in a nursing home, or managing a chronic condition in our own homes—at some of our most vulnerable moments—nurses are the healthcare providers we are most likely to encounter, spend the greatest amount of time with, and be dependent upon for our recovery" (IOM, 2004a, p. *ix*). Following a review of the clinical work environment, the report discusses designs for a work environment in which nurses can provide safer, higher quality patient care. It explores the nursing shortage, healthcare errors, patient safety risk factors, the central role of the nurse in patient safety, and work environment threats to patient safety. Like earlier quality reports, it calls for a change from blaming individuals for errors to greater consideration of the many system factors that influence outcomes, such as equipment failures, inadequate staff training, lack of clear supervision and direction, inadequate staffing levels, and so on. To make the necessary improvements will require a transformation of the work environment.

It is first important to understand how work is done in order to build patient safety measures into the nursing work environment. The report identifies six major concerns for direct care in nursing (IOM, 2004a, pp. 91–100).

1. *Monitoring patient status or surveillance*, which, according to the report, is different from assessment. Surveillance is defined as "purposeful and *ongoing* acquisition, interpretation, and synthesis of patient data for clinical decision-making" (McCloskey & Bulechek, 2000, p. 629).
2. *Physiologic therapy*, the most common visible interventions that nurses perform.
3. *Helping patients compensate for loss of function*; many related activities are performed by unlicensed assistive personnel (UAPs) under the direction of registered nurses (RNs), but RNs do this as well.
4. *Providing emotional support,* critical for patients and their families.
5. *Education for patients and families*, which has become more difficult for practicing nurses to provide because of work conditions and the staffing shortage.
6. *Integration and coordination of care*: patients' needs are complex, and care is complex, often resulting in multiple forms of care provided by multiple providers. There is a high risk of failure in communication and inadequate collaboration, both of which increase the risk of errors. There is a critical need for interdisciplinary teams.

The report recommends (1) adopting transformational leadership and evidence-based management, (2) maximizing the capability of the workforce, and (3) creating and sustaining cultures of safety. These are elaborated in Appendix H.

In line with this report, the Institute for Healthcare Improvement's (IHI) 100,000 Lives Campaign aims to create a safety net for patients. As of November 2005, approximately 2,800 hospitals had signed on to this initiative (Scalise, 2005). Another example is ANA's initiative on "Safe Handling." The University of Oklahoma Health Sciences Center College of Nursing is one of the participants, as is the University of Oklahoma Medical Center. ANA's call for action *Handle with Care* asked schools of nursing to partner with clinical agencies and other professional organizations to develop safer techniques for handling, lifting, and moving patients in order to keep nurses safe from back injuries and other musculoskeletal injuries. This curriculum also involves the use of lifting equipment that can be obtained through grants for nursing skills labs. Reducing such injuries means healthier nurses, better workplace environments, and retention of staff, particularly as patients have gotten more obese and their conditions have made lifting necessary.

## *Health Professions Education Report*

### Health Professions Education: A Bridge to Quality (2003)

Education of health professionals is viewed as a bridge to quality care. The discussion centers on education and the need to have qualified, competent staff to improve health care, and concludes that health professions education needs to change to meet the growing demands of current and future healthcare systems. The report clearly states that the goal of health professions education should be outcome-based education. Health care in the United States requires changes to improve healthcare quality and safety, and these changes should consider outcomes.

These recommendations are hardly surprising. However, the report makes clear that health professions education has not kept current with healthcare needs, evidence-based practice, technology, diversity changes, and leadership requirements, putting it even further behind in light of newer recommendations. *The Essentials of Baccalaureate Education for Professional Nursing Practice* (AACN, 1998) includes, to some extent, all the core competencies recommended in the IOM report. "Yet the current challenges before us are twofold: to determine why the current workforce of baccalaureate-prepared nurses is not fully actualizing the IOM core competencies and to consider ways to strengthen nursing curricula to better educate nurses" (Long, 2003, pp. 259–260).

The five core competencies recommended for implementation by all organizations involved in the education of healthcare professionals are:

1. Provide patient-centered care—focus on the patient rather than disease or the clinician.
2. Work in interdisciplinary teams—utilize the best healthcare professionals for the needs of the patient and work together to accomplish effective patient care outcomes.
3. Employ evidence-based practice—integrate best research results, clinical expertise, and patient values to make patient care decisions.
4. Apply quality improvement (QI)—not only apply QI but make it effective.
5. Utilize informatics—apply it to reduction of errors, management of knowledge and information, decision-making, and communication (IOM, 2003e, pp. 49–63).

*Health Professions Education: A Bridge to Quality* outlines some strategies to build these competencies. These strategies and recommendations are found in Appendix I.

## *Summary*

The major IOM reports from the Quality Healthcare Initiative provide important data and recommendations that should help to improve healthcare quality and safety nationally. The reports begin with a critical examination of healthcare safety and quality, and proceed to:

1. Develop frameworks and terminology for data analysis, action plans, and reporting mechanisms,
2. Define the role of leadership, particularly the role of government,
3. Explore critical issues related to public health and diversity,
4. Specify the priorities of quality improvement initiatives,
5. Analyze the nursing workplace, and
6. Examine health professions education and identify core competencies for all health professions.

# Part 2

# Strategies for Nursing Education

Improvement in healthcare goes hand-in-hand with improved health professions education (IOM, 2003a). The IOM reports indicate that much needs to be done; however, the reports will not mean anything to nursing education unless the recommendations and findings are integrated into educational systems. There is a "quality chasm" between the "ivory tower" of healthcare education and the healthcare delivery system. The IOM reports clearly show the gaps in education still present several years after the first reports were published. "Education for health professions is in need of a major overhaul. Clinical education simply has not kept pace with or been responsive enough to shifting patient demographics and desires, changing health system expectations, evolving practice requirements and staffing arrangements, new information, a focus on improving quality, or new technologies" (IOM, 2001b as cited in IOM, 2003a, p. 1). Part 2 proposes nursing education strategies to close these gaps.

## A Challenge and Some Q&A for Nursing Educators

When Tim Porter O'Grady addressed an American Academy of Nursing (AAN) leadership conference in November 2004, he stated, "we are never going to combat the nursing shortage with increasing numbers because we have the wrong people doing the wrong things." Likewise, nursing faculty may be teaching the wrong things and emphasizing the wrong skills. This is a challenge for all schools of nursing; they need to critically examine what is taught and how it contributes to the education of safe practitioners. Many questions need answers:

- *Is it still necessary to teach a foundations course to ease students into their clinical skills or to teach health assessment as a separate nursing course?* Similar courses are also taught in allied health, medical school, and other health-related disciplines. Health and physical assessment could be taught across disciplines if health professions faculty and administrators would stop arguing about head counts and who gets the tuition dollar, and instead work out a business model that dispenses with these antiquated rules. This content could be modularized and taught mostly in a virtual mode. If competency-based evaluation is the focus, once the skill is mastered the student moves on. Today, many excellent online materials are offered by textbook publishers, who have the financial resources to develop sophisticated graphics, audios, and simulations that can be used for content such as health assessment and pharmacology. Why should nursing education reinvent this content or try to develop new material? Why not collaborate with other health professions educators, businesses, and publishers? With this material, skills could then be reinforced in the simulation lab and clinical settings.

- *What should be emphasized in either the classroom or clinical?* Critical thinking, rationales behind decisions, and evidence-based practice (EPB) need more emphasis. How more content can be added to the curriculum is a legitimate question. However, it is more instructive to ask:
  - Why do faculty feel as if they must try to teach everything?
  - What is covered?
  - What really needs to be covered?
  - Are schools driven by what individual faculty members want to present rather than what is really required to practice?
  - When are we going overboard and losing focus?
  - When should faculty expect students to master the content and then work with students to apply that knowledge (critical thinking, EBP, and so on)?
- *How can clinical rotations be enhanced so that they maximize learning experiences?* Many faculty complain that not enough time is devoted to clinical experiences without considering when faculty last evaluated how clinical time was actually used. They should be willing to step back from the way things have always been done and consider new approaches to clinical experiences. It may be more effective to use clinical facilities for several intensive weeks rather than intersperse clinical with classroom experiences. This way the students have a better chance to see the results of their care planning and continuity of care, and to gain the skills that make them feel more confident. "Visiting" clinical settings has not proven helpful. Students need to spend extended time there to better understand the work environment, professionalism, and the complexities of patient care. It is difficult to cultivate more team experiences in only a few hours, maybe two days a week.

McBride (2005) suggests that to achieve our goal nursing education must recognize that health care's paradigm has shifted; the IOM reports show that informatics must be at the core of healthcare systems. McBride goes on to say, "the emphasis on the nursing process and the nurse–patient relationship may have inadvertently made us less prepared for today's emphasis on outcomes and the obligation we have to transform our work settings into learning organizations. Our pride in being 'high touch' may get in the way of seeing opportunities in telehealth" (p. 28). The shift in paradigms is "from process orientation (what the professional is doing) to outcomes orientation (the value of what the professional is doing); from focus on provider–patient relationship to focus on the work setting as a learning organization; from *do no harm* as an individual responsibility to safety as a system concern; from caregiving that is time- and place-bound to caregiving with time and place limitations removed; from focus of care that emphasizes patient compliance to focus of care that emphasizes best practices; from workarounds being the norm to crucial conversations being the norm; from decision-making based on training and experience to evidence-based decision-making; from organizations that encourage professional silos to organizations that encourage interdisciplinary collaboration; from seeking cost reductions to continuously decreasing waste; from emphasis on discharge planning to emphasis on lifestyle change" (p. 22).

These are some of the more general nursing education issues related to quality. It is critical for nursing faculty to respond effectively to these IOM reports and consult with their counterparts in practice to arrive at measures that will improve care through more effective teaching and learning.

## *A Nursing Response to the IOM Reports: Nursing Education Strategies*

All health professionals should be educated to deliver patient-centered care as members of an interdisciplinary team, emphasizing evidence-based practice, quality improvement approaches, and informatics (IOM, 2003a, p. 3). Nursing education must adapt to the changing demographics of the patient population, integrate technologies, and meet critical competencies identified in the recommendations.

### React to the Shifting Demographics of the Patient Population

Americans are older than ever, living with multiple comorbidities and chronic health needs. The other end of the life span is also at increasing risk, with a population of children who before the age of 10 are experiencing comorbidities such as hypertension, diabetes, and obesity; furthermore, many women are delaying childbearing well into their forties, which may lead to complications during pregnancy and for the newborn. These demographics indicate that long-term health care will require a care delivery system that can handle this growing complexity. Since these are major shifts from the patient pool of the past, healthcare professionals need education that prepares them to handle complex healthcare problems in a more efficient, safer way.

At the same time, the population is becoming more diverse. Cultural beliefs and values must be integrated into teaching health, yet most programs gloss over cultural competence. The challenge is not to add content but to integrate content, and to keep it current with safety, quality, and diversity issues. This will become part of the routine learning experience when students in the clinical setting are expected to include the demographics and cultural backgrounds of their patients in clinical conferences, address them in patient care plans, and incorporate them into written assignments.

### Recognize and Integrate Technology Competencies into the Nursing Curriculum

Informatics must become a curricular thread throughout educational levels. Care plans must reflect EMR charting, and teaching should reinforce the process in both its nursing and medical aspects. Students then need an opportunity to apply this informatics knowledge in the clinical areas. In the classroom, students need to see examples of physician order entry systems, pharmacy orders, and electronic medical records. These technology skills then become part of the critical skills that compose nursing education expectations and competencies. Technology competencies and a working knowledge of Systematic Nomenclature of Medicine (SNOMED), International Classification of Diseases Ninth Revision (ICD9), and Current Procedural Terminology (CPT) coding are essential; the nurse must understand how a uniform language makes nursing actions retrievable and how services are reimbursed. At the undergraduate level this information may be limited to an appreciation of the coding systems, not the practice of coding, whereas advanced practice nursing students need to know about the application of coding.

EBP should be more than educators citing studies in various classes. In exercises students should gather evidence and critically review studies much as the research process that has been taught in the past, but now students should be asked to determine what level of evidence supports the nursing interventions that they implement. Students may work on such evidence-based projects instead of developing a research proposal or, at the master's level, writing a thesis. Where there is an evidence-based practice center, undergraduates can learn how to glean information from the literature and evaluate its credibility, and then write a short report on the process. This exercise allows students to learn how a discipline examines evidence, how little evidence there is to support many nursing interventions, the need for more rigorous studies, and the use of computer skills to gather information quickly and condense it to a usable form. Informatics is a critical tool for students as they learn to apply EBP.

Quality improvement exercises are also a necessary part of the papers that students write. Faculty should review current assignments to determine how they reflect QI and how students can better apply it to their practice. Students first need to understand the ANA National Quality Database, the issues that ANA and AAN are investigating through the interdisciplinary group the National Quality Forum (NQF), and how the ANA Report Card is now being used by JCAHO. These quality indicators have been linked to patient safety outcomes in such areas as medication errors and falls, and they are being integrated into electronic medical records and physician order entry systems. So it seems reasonable that students and faculty apply these same measures to nursing education.

This material could be added to the admittedly bulging curriculum the same way that AACN essentials are incorporated. Once educators agree that this is essential content, it will be integrated. This also calls for a careful examination of what is currently being taught, with consideration of how the curriculum can fit into a quality framework. A course called Health II that focuses on immune disorders could include cancer as an example of a failure of the immune system. The genetic aspects of these problems would be taught with additional coverage of the quality indicators and EBP that are most appropriate for one or two sample cases. Faculty and students could work through the cases using a POES and EMR process—this could be done with computer screen shots in the classroom to demonstrate how errors might occur or be prevented by override systems to stop certain drugs from being ordered beyond normal limits or with a potential interaction with another drug. This case experience would emphasize technology integration, informatics, quality, and the uniform language of the discipline all in one learning experience. This is not really adding content; it is merely presenting it so that students acquire not just information but insight into how it is applied.

Much more teaching could be centered on case-based, problem-based learning. Every disease does not need to be taught, though frequently efforts are made to do this. If several diseases are used as examples, it will allow more time to include other content such as cultural values and beliefs. For example, discuss diet alterations necessary in cancer treatment with an understanding of Muslim dietary beliefs (patient-centered care), the effects of age and living conditions on the health promotion of the individual and family from a team approach (interdisciplinary care), the impact of healthcare costs and coverage or reimbursement of services, and safety and QI. Present evidence to support the plan (EBP). This moves the lecture from a laundry list to an application of knowledge, provides students with an up-to-date framework for learning that can then be applied to other diseases, and incorporates critical new concepts into the curriculum.

### Conduct Root Cause Analysis of Errors

Students should be asked to find errors and breaches of quality care. They should then use root cause analysis to determine at what level the error occurred. Whether it happened at the point of care or at the system level will determine the steps needed to improve care in the future (quality improvement). This teaches not only the nursing process but the process of root cause analysis and the use of informatics to render and evaluate care (informatics).

## *General Nursing Education Issues*

Like IOM, nursing education recognizes the need for competency-based education and is moving in this direction. IOM's core competencies are not unknown to nursing education, either, although we need to do much more in that regard. Here are further examples of how nursing is responding to issues raised by the IOM reports.

## New Pathways

AACN is working to create new educational pathways to provide the new level of knowledge that providers need. The two main initiatives are the Clinical Nurse Leader (CNL) and the Doctor of Nursing Practice (DNP).

### *Clinical Nurse Leader*

The CNL was conceptualized in 2003 and is now in the pilot stage. A summit meeting of 140 clinical agencies and 80 nursing schools, funded by AHRQ, was held in July 2003. Each educational institution had to have at least one clinical partner to be a part of the pilot; they are in the process of creating curricula and determining quality outcome measures (AACN, 2005a). This realizes the IOM recommendation to launch summits with healthcare organizations, educational institutions, and funding agencies.

The CNL role is described as "a leader in the healthcare delivery system across all settings in which health care is delivered, not just the acute care setting. The implementation of the CNL role, however, will vary across settings. The role is not one of administration or management. The CNL assumes accountability for client care outcomes through the assimilation and application of research-based information to design, implement, and evaluate client plans of care. The CNL is a provider and a manager of care at the point of care to individuals, cohorts, or populations. The CNL designs, implements, and evaluates client care by coordinating, delegating and supervising the care provided by the healthcare team, including licensed nurses, technicians, and other health professionals" (AACN, 2005a, http://www.aacn.nche.edu/CNL/).

This role is viewed as the integrator that keeps patients and families from being overlooked by the seemingly broken healthcare system. It requires knowledge of financial models, justifying healthcare costs, obtaining reimbursement for services, health policy needs, ethics, resource management, and use of technology, just to name a few skills. While some of these activities are not new to nursing, what is new is that this role is at the point of care and is not a manager role.

The CNL is unit-based, hence not as easily cut from the budget as the system-based Clinical Nurse Specialist (CNS). Being unit-based and population-based, the CNL can move from unit to unit as changes occur in healthcare delivery. In many respects this role is the case management role—the overseer of care coordination. While AACN recommends implementation at the master's level, some of these skills and content can be included in BSN programs. BSN-level graduates in rural states may find themselves Chief Nursing Officers very quickly, or at least nurse managers who need to understand the same principles as the CNL.

### *Doctor of Nursing Practice*

The Doctor of Nursing Practice or DNP evolved from seminal work of an AACN Task Force that met at a 2003 summit with the National Organization of Nurse Practitioner Faculties (NONPF). This summit brought together educational institutions, clinical agencies, regulatory and certifying bodies, and other nursing organizations, once again in line with one of the IOM recommendations. In 2004, AACN hosted a reaction panel composed of medicine, academic health science, healthcare administration, higher education, and law to discuss the need for and implementation of DNP-level education (AACN, 2005a).

Practice in the DNP program represents any facet of practice, including nursing administration. It grew out of the perception that master's level nurses needed more advanced diagnostic and assessment skills, and that the years of education were not commensurate with the degree granted (AACN, 2005b). It was also acknowledged that not all nurses wanted a research doctorate so much as a clinically focused degree. The length of most master's programs was nearer that of doctoral programs in other professions, such as pharmacy and allied health. Again with a view to the IOM emphasis on quality of care, patient safety, and interdisciplinary work, AACN has specified seven essential educational areas for the DNP: (1) scientific underpinnings for practice; (2) advanced nursing practice; (3) organization and system leadership and management, quality improvement, and system thinking; (4) analytic methodologies related to the evaluation of practice and the application of evidence for practice; (5) utilization of technology and information for the improvement and transformation of health care; (6) health policy development, implementation, and evaluation; and (7) interdisciplinary collaboration for improving patient and population healthcare outcomes (AACN, 2005c, http://www.aacn.nche.edu/Education/index.htm). This doctorate is considered a terminal degree, and the graduate is expected to provide visionary leadership that integrates systems knowledge and influences policy to promote best practices in the clinical arena. This person is also expected to participate in EBP and to work with nurses to design research utilization projects. The objectives and curriculum for this pathway at the University of South Carolina College of Nursing include:

- Manage health care of individuals and communities in complex healthcare systems.
- Conduct research utilization studies to innovate practice.
- Influence healthcare policy at the local, state, and national levels.
- Assume leadership roles in health care.

Tables 2-1, 2-2, and 2-3 break down the curriculum for students entering the program from different educational backgrounds.

### Centers of Excellence

Another consequence of the IOM reports is a greater need for national recognition of excellence in nursing education. The Centers of Excellence in the Magnet Hospital Recognition Program for healthcare organizations can serve as a model for Centers of Excellence in Nursing Education. Just as hospitals that have attained Magnet status have used this recognition to attract the best nurses, using something similar to the

**TABLE 2-1 Pre-DNP Curriculum For Non-BSN Prepared Students Admitted Prior To Fall 2005**

| *Course Number* | *Course Title* | *Cr Hr* | *Non-BSN/ w Other Degree* | *Non-BSN/ w ADN* |
|---|---|---|---|---|
| NURS 309 | Nursing Health Assessment | 3 | X | |
| NURS 310 | Clinical Therapeutics | 3 | X | |
| NURS 315 | Nursing Adults I | 5 | X | |
| NURS 317 | Psychosocial Pathology | 2 | X | X |
| NURS 320 | Clinical Reasoning | 3 | X | X |
| NURS 322 | Nursing Adults II | 5 | X | |
| NURS 323 | Nursing of Older Adults | 5 | X | |
| NURS 414 | Nursing of Childbearing Families | 5 | X | |
| NURS 415 | Nursing of Childrearing Families | 5 | X | |
| NURS 701a | Preceptored Clinical Practice | 2 | X | X |
| NURS 701b | Preceptored Clinical Practice | 2 | X | X |
| *Total Credit Hours* | | | 40 | 9 |

Forces of Magnetism (see below) to recruit and retain superior faculty and students will revitalize nursing education and create an air of competition and a sense of pride in the end products of nursing schools—their graduates.

The National League for Nursing (NLN) established one method for identifying schools of nursing that excel through their Centers for Excellence in Nursing Education Program, established in 2003 (http://www.nln.org). This program recognizes schools of nursing that demonstrate sustained, evidence-based, and substantive innovation in one of three ways: (1) enhance student learning and professional development, (2) promote ongoing faculty development, and (3) advance nursing

**TABLE 2-2 Pre-DNP Curriculum For Non-BSN Prepared Students Beginning Fall 2005**

| *Course Number* | *Course Title* | *Cr Hr* | *Non-BSN/ w Other Degree* | *Non-BSN/ w ADN* |
|---|---|---|---|---|
| NURS 311 | Introduction to Health Assessment | 2 | X | |
| NURS 312 | Foundations of Nursing Practice | 4 | X | |
| NURS 314 | Clinical Reasoning in Nursing Practice | 2 | X | X |
| NURS 317 | Psychosocial Pathology | 3 | X | X |
| NURS 319 | Health Across the Life Span | 3 | X | |
| NURS 411 | Psychiatric/Mental Health Nursing | 5 | X | |
| NURS 412 | Acute Care Nursing of Adults I | 5 | X | |
| NURS 422 | Acute Care Nursing of Adults II | 5 | X | |
| NURS 424 | Maternal/Newborn Nursing | 3 | X | |
| NURS 425 | Nursing of Children and Families | 3 | X | |
| NURS 491 | Community and Environmental Assessment | 1 | X | X |
| NURS 432 | Adult Health Nursing Preceptorship | 4 | X | X |
| NURS 433 | Nursing Leadership and Management Preceptorship | 4 | X | X |
| *Total Credit Hours* | | | 44 | 14 |

**TABLE 2-3 DNP Curriculum Plan for BSN to DNP Students***

| *I: Research/Theory Core (taken by all DNP students)* | *II: Leadership/Policy Core (taken by all DNP students)* | *III: Advanced Practice Core (taken by all DNP students)* | *IV: Area of Specialization (select at least one)* |
|---|---|---|---|
| NURS 700 Theoretical and Conceptual Foundation for Nursing (3) | EPID 700 Introduction to Epidemiology (3) | HGEN 700 Medical Genetics for Healthcare Professionals (3) | **Acute Care Clinical Nurse Specialist:** NURS 725 (2), 727 (3), 750 (3), 786 (4), and 6 credit hours electives upon advisement. |
| NURS 737 Seminar on Advanced Practice Roles (1) | NURS 708 Conceptual Basis for Family and Community Health Nursing (3) | NURS 702 Pharmacologic Management in Primary Care (3) | **Acute Care Nurse Practitioner:** NURS 786 (5), 787 (5) and 8 credit hours electives upon advisement. |
| BIOS 700 Introduction to Biostatistics (3) | NURS 720 Public Health Residency (Program Planning and Evaluation) (3) | NURS 704 Advanced Health Assessment (3) | **Community/Public Health Nursing Administration:** NURS 716 (3), 720 (3), HSPM 700 (3) and 9 credit hours by advisement. |
| BIOS 757 Statistics II (EDRM 711 or STATS 701) (3) | NURS 734 Conceptual Basis of Health Systems (3) | NURS 707 Advanced Pathophysiology for Nurses (3) | **Community Health Promotion and Education:** NURS 716 (3), 720 (3), HPEB 700 (3) and 9 credit hours by advisement. |
| NURS 790 Research Methods for Nursing (3) | NURS 735 Case Management (1) | NURS 718 Diagnostic Interpretation and Therapeutic Modalities (3) | **Gerontologic Clinical Nurse Specialist:** NURS 733 (1), 752 (3), 753 (3), 754 (3), 755 (3), 756 (3), and 2 credit hours electives upon advisement. |
| NURS 821 Research Utilization Preparation (6 total) | NURS 738/HSPM730 Financing of Health care (3) | NURS 731 Management of Psychiatric Health Problems in Primary Care (3) | **Nursing Administration:** NURS 740 (3), 741 (3), 742 (3), 781 (3), HSPM 712 (3), MGMT 770 (3). |
| | NURS 779/HSPM 711 Health Politics (3) | NURS 793 Advanced Practice Clinical Practicum (3) | **Occupational/Environmental Health Nursing:** NURS 716 (3), 720 (3), ENHS 660 (3) and 9 credit hours by advisement. |
| | NURS 794/ PHIL710/DMED 620/SOWK 753/PUBH 710 Ethics and the Health Sciences (3) | NURS 820 Nursing Leadership Residency (3) | **Primary Care Nurse Practitioner, Adult:** 705 (3) 722 (3), and 12 credit hours by advisement. |
| | | | **Primary Care Nurse Practitioner, Family:** NURS 705 (3), 706 (3), 722 (3), and 9 credit hours by advisement. |
| | | | **Primary Care Nurse Practitioner, Gerontologic:** NURS 705 (3), 722 (3), 753 (3), and 9 credit hours by advisement. |
| | | | **Primary Care Nurse Practitioner, Pediatric:** NURS 706 (3), 710 (3), 722 (3), and 9 credit hours by advisement. |
| | | | **Psychiatric Nurse Practitioner/Specialist, Adult:** NURS 705 (3), 722 (3), 732 (3), 733 (1), 735 (2), and 6 credit hours electives by advisement. |
| | | | **Psychiatric Nurse Practitioner/Specialist, Child/Adolescent:** NURS 706 (3), 710 (3), 722 (3), 732 (3), 733 (1), 735 (2), and 3 credit hours electives by advisement. |
| | | | **Psychiatric Clinical Nurse Specialist:** NURS 732 (3), 733 (1), 735 (2), 789 (3), and 9 credit hours electives by advisement. |
| | | | **School Health Nursing:** NURS 716 (3), 720 (3), HPEB 720 (3) and 9 credit hours by advisement. |
| | | | **Women's Health Nurse Practitioner:** NURS 705 (3), 722 (3), 739 (3), 776 (4), and 5 credit hours electives upon advisement. |
| 19 Credits | 22 Credits | 24 Credits | 18 Credits |

*For MSN-prepared students, up to 50% of required course work may be waived if equivalent courses were completed in the student's master's curriculum. Courses with non-nursing prefixes are either cross-listed with courses in other disciplines or used as an alternative equivalency.

*Reproduced with permission of ****

education research. Each is critical, but to advance nursing education, a school will need to excel in more than one area. The goals of the NLN recognition program are:

- To encourage faculty to continually improve their schools,
- To encourage research in nursing education,
- To facilitate discussions among faculty, students, graduates, and employers about excellence in nursing education and how to promote it,
- To encourage the development of innovative schools that attract and retain highly qualified students and faculty,
- To reshape nursing education based on the application of evidence from research in practice and education, and
- To support public policies that benefit nursing education, support nursing education research, and promote excellence in nursing education (http://www.nln.org).

### Schools of Nursing and Forces of Magnetism

The Magnet Program and its Forces of Magnetism (McClure & Hinshaw, 2002) can be applied to schools of nursing and assist in developing Centers of Excellence in Nursing Education. These Forces of Magnetism incorporate all three NLN areas of focus. A school of nursing applying for recognition would complete a critical self-study of operations, business practices, outcomes, patient satisfaction, clinical agency evaluations, and faculty and staff satisfaction. It would also need to provide documentation of examination of teaching and learning principles in the context of educational research. Partnerships with hospitals and other colleges across disciplines are essential to determine fields for research to support best practices. Databases will support analysis to discern what promotes student excellence and graduates who not only pass licensure or specialty certification examinations but render effective care; track attrition and retention rates; and document faculty productivity. AACN's 2004 annual report notes that while enrollments are up in all levels of nursing education, graduation rates for masters have declined 2.5% and doctorates 9.9% (AACN, 2005a). The factors behind this decline need to be examined. The workplace environment and factors of morale, productivity, attrition, and retention should be applied to the college's faculty and staff. Both faculty and staff have to support a more consumer-driven environment that places the student in the center. Excellence requires that both incentives for productive staff members and measures to deal with unsatisfactory employees be examined. The forces of magnetism that draw students, faculty, and staff to institutions should be fostered.

Once the critical analysis has been completed, action plans that are living and not stagnant are vital to achieve excellence. This movement in education is embryonic, but if it catches on like Magnet Recognition for hospitals, it will become a credential that all educational institutions covet. While today there is one example from NLN, similar programs are bound to evolve from other organizations such as AACN. The display, Forces of Magnetism, on pages 22 and 23 presents these forces as they could be adapted to nursing education.

### Reviewing and Updating Nursing Curriculum

Nursing educators must also find a more effective method for curriculum review and update. They must abandon the old processes that take years. With the frequent changes in knowledge and today's ability to access knowledge quickly, taking years to accomplish updates will not serve the students, or their employers when they graduate. Early in the review process, make the curriculum something the faculty own and thus feel committed to implementing. There can be no sacred areas of content that cannot be touched. Without a doubt, nurse educators cannot keep adding content, so it will take flexibility and willingness to consider all content open to change. Barriers that make faculty think they cannot add more content include:

- Repeated content (e.g., students have taken pathophysiology, yet this is repeated in adult health content such as cardiac disease or diabetes),
- Thinking that everything must be covered in class instead of expecting students to come to class prepared,
- Faculty adding content that is not officially approved or monitored,
- Inadequate review of textbooks when reading assignments are made (students cannot distinguish "nice to know" from "need to know," making reading assignments too long),
- Too little expectation that students know and apply information from previous courses,
- Little or ineffective use of simulation,
- Ignoring adult principles of education,
- Limited use of online methods to cover content that can then be applied in the classroom, seminars, or practica, or used as standalone courses, and
- Lack of innovative methods for integrating online materials.

A rich source of information for healthcare providers and nurse educators is the annual National Healthcare Quality Report, as well as the annual report on disparities in healthcare delivery. Curricula do not always consider the real status or multiple dimensions of health care, partly because these data have not been easy to access or even to isolate. Data that are collected are often related to a single institution, a geographic region, or a specific disease entity and not reflective of a national perspective. Sometimes faculty have just preferred to do it the way it has usually been done—maybe changing some terminology but still intent on the same healthcare issues. Granted, many of these issues will probably show up in a National Quality Report, but new issues may arise.

Schools of nursing do not change easily or quickly. Some faculty may not see the connection between IOM reports and education, and may view the report as related

**Forces of Magnetisim**

*Quality of nursing leadership.* Nursing education leaders are perceived as knowledgeable, strong risk-takers who follow an articulated philosophy in the day-to-day operations of the school of nursing. Nursing education leaders also convey a strong sense of advocacy and support on behalf of the faculty, staff, and students.

*Organizational structure.* The organizational structure of the school of nursing is characterized as flat, rather that tall, and faculty decision-making prevails. There is strong faculty representation evident in the organizational committee structure. The nursing leader serves at the executive level of the organization, and as the chief of the nursing school.

*Management style.* Nursing education leaders use a participative management style, incorporating feedback from faculty, staff, and students at all levels of the organization. Feedback is encouraged and valued. Nurses serving in leadership positions are visible, accessible, and committed to communicating effectively with faculty, staff, and students.

*Personnel policies and programs.* Salaries and benefits are competitive. Flexible and effective staffing models and teaching assignments are used. Personnel policies are created with faculty and staff involvement, and significant administrative, teaching, and clinical promotional opportunities exist.

*Professional models of care.* Models of teaching are used that give faculty the responsibility and authority for developing and implementing a curriculum that addresses current healthcare needs and delivery issues. Faculty are accountable for their own practice, and faculty practice is supported, such as clinical, administrative, and other types of practice as methods of increasing faculty expertise and partnership with the healthcare delivery system.

*Quality of care.* Faculty perceive that they are providing high-quality nursing education. Providing quality education is seen as an organizational priority as well, and the faculty serving in leadership positions are viewed as responsible for ensuring an environment in which high-quality education can be provided.

(*continued*)

only to the practice area. For faculty who do wish to change the curriculum to include such material, it is not easy. Curricular changes often take on issues of academic freedom, time for more content, and faculty workloads, and ignore how essential this content is to nurses. Furthermore, curricular changes may take years. The key for success today is to make change happen more quickly so that students are prepared: keeping up with new healthcare concerns is critical. A curriculum framework that allows for change as need arises is imperative. Sources such as the National Healthcare Quality Report, IOM reports, and *Healthy People 2010* will provide more direc-

*Quality improvement.* Quality improvement activities are viewed as educational. All faculty participate in the quality improvement process and perceive the process as one that improves the quality of education delivered within the organization.

*Consultation and resources.* Adequate consultation and other human resources are available. Knowledgeable experts are available and are used. In addition, peer support is given within the school.

*Autonomy.* Faculty are permitted and expected to teach autonomously, consistent with professional standards, but also expected to work as team members. Independent judgment is expected to be exercised within the context of an interdisciplinary approach to patient care and teaching.

*Community and the hospital.* Schools of nursing that are best able to recruit and retain faculty also maintain a strong community presence. A community presence is seen in a variety of ongoing, long-term outreach programs. These outreach programs result in the school of nursing being perceived as a strong, positive, and productive corporate citizen.

*Nurses as teachers.* Nursing faculty are permitted and expected to practice and to act as role models for students.

*Image of nursing.* The school of nursing is viewed as integral part of the university and healthcare services within the community. The services provided by the faculty are characterized as essential by other members of the healthcare team.

*Interdisciplinary relationship.* The school of nursing applies an interdisciplinary approach to teaching, working with other disciplines in developing interdisciplinary content and a learning experience that facilitates student learning and develops interdisciplinary team skills.

*Professional development.* Significant emphasis is placed on faculty and student orientation, faculty development, formal education, and career development. Personal and professional growth and development are valued.

Source: Adapted from McClure & Hinshaw, 2002, pp. 106–107.

tion to the review and change process. Course descriptions and objectives that allow for this approach will be required. Schools of nursing that choose not to do this will not produce the best-qualified frontline practitioners. Nurse researchers typically approach research with an open mind and look for new needs; nurse educators must do this also. They must be able not only to use information from the Quality Report but also to connect that information to practice—understanding what is occurring in healthcare settings, how this affects what should be taught, and the implications of the Quality Report. Appendix L provides critical information from the IOM reports that might be used to develop a curriculum schema.

There is no doubt that nurses today are inundated with crucial information. Textbooks are important, but learning should not end there. Faculty and students can benefit from critical updates about important aspects of health care and needed improvements. This should be true on the undergraduate level as well as the graduate level. The Internet has opened doors to information that once was either unavailable or difficult to find.

Greater use of online education is a given in many schools today. How it is used, the quality of the courses, and how the outcomes are evaluated are all important questions. Students are more and more involved in information technology (IT) and expect schools and faculty to use IT. Some programs blend online education with face-to-face education either in the classroom, virtual, or in clinical. This is exemplified by a partnership between a for-profit company Orbis Education and the University of Oklahoma Health Sciences Center College of Nursing (OUCON). Experience in creating interactive online courses coupled with the ability to attract clinical partners for practica experience forges a mutually beneficial partnership. The advantage to the healthcare partner is that the students only do rotations in one healthcare organization (HCO) and thus are recruited to stay there after graduation. The school of nursing can add faculty and students without being dependent on state or private revenue, provide quality just-in-time education, increase accessibility of the programs, and use the technology to mentor novice teachers in how to teach both online and in a clinical setting.

These innovative models have advantages for nursing programs, students, and HCOs. Students are better able to adjust their school schedule to personal needs when they can "attend" class when it fits their schedule. Students still have face-to-face contact with faculty either in periodic meetings, seminars, and conferences or in clinical. Scheduling classes and use of space for classes is simplified. Students accept responsibility for their own learning. Online courses provide more opportunities for interactive as opposed to lecture-based learning, using cases, interactive gaming techniques, and much more, but this does require financial, design, and technology resources.

An important step in answering IOM's call for better collaboration was the 2005 conference on Transforming Health Professional Education, led by Joint Commission Resources (a JCAHO affiliate), but cosponsored by organizations representing nursing, medical, pharmacy, and health administration education and some healthcare organizations. The goal was to begin an interdisciplinary dialogue to improve health professions education, with topics such as what needs to be redesigned, what models of change exist, and how to create a learning continuum.

One clear theme was the need for more interdisciplinary learning, and much needs to be done to accomplish this. Nurse educators need to assume a major role in response to this conference by actively pursuing opportunities to improve. Healthcare professions students should be included in clinical activities such as attending teams, grand rounds presentations, specialty weekly conferences, patient rounds, and any clinical activity where patient care is discussed. More interdisciplinary courses are needed. Some might focus only on interdisciplinary work teams, with content such as advantages and disadvantages of working together; roles and scope of practice; improvement of collaboration, coordination, and communication; impact on the patient; leadership and followership; and impact on safety and quality.

Getting nursing, medical, pharmacy, allied health, and any other health professions students who may be located in the academic center into a course that asks them to learn about teams and openly discuss these issues can be a significant first step. Other courses might concentrate on cases, health assessment, or simulation labs where teams of students respond to simulated scenarios and debrief afterward. An interdisciplinary course might focus on safety and quality, where students form teams, select a safety or quality problem, analyze it, develop resolutions, and then determine how outcomes would be evaluated. This type of course will naturally include many of the issues described earlier, where students explore what it means to be on a team. Here they would experience this fully as they work to reach an outcome.

# Part 3

# Incorporating the Core Competencies in Nursing Education

The strategies for integrating safety and quality into nursing education are based on the five core competencies found in *Health Professions Education* (IOM, 2003): (1) provide patient-centered care, (2) work in interdisciplinary teams, (3) employ evidence-based practice, (4) apply quality improvement, and (5) utilize information. The complementary topic of informational and organizational transparency is also addressed.

## Provide Patient-Centered Care

*Identify, respect, and care about patients' differences, values, preferences, and expressed needs; relieve pain and suffering; coordinate continuous care; listen to, clearly inform, communicate with, and educate patients; share decision-making and management; and continuously advocate disease prevention, wellness, and promotion of healthy lifestyles, including a focus on population health* (IOM, 2003, p. 4).

Patient-centered care puts the focus back on the patient and family instead of the health professionals. For example, instead of having the patient move from room to room to see different specialists, the health professionals come to the patient.

### Decentralized and Fragmented Care

Students experience fragmented care with their patients but may not recognize it, or if they do recognize it, are often frustrated by it. Asking students how it felt when they first entered the healthcare setting as a student—their confusion, inability to know what is going on, uncertainty of who staff were and what were the expectations, communication, and so on—can help them better appreciate what patients may be feeling. Many students worry about "drive-through health care." When a test is delayed or postponed because someone did not order it, how does the patient feel and react, and what impact does this have on patient care when the student's well-planned schedule for care is no longer well planned? If students can understand their own feelings, they can be asked: "Well, if you feel this way, how do you think the patient feels?"

Fragmented care is everywhere. Ask students to name examples, then ask them to think of practical solutions. Iatrogenic injury can be related to fragmented care, and students need to consider how this might occur. Provide specific examples from different healthcare settings such as acute care, emergency room, ambulatory care, and home care, so that students can gain an understanding of how fragmented care might occur and how the setting may influence results.

Discuss the implications of decentralization and fragmentation as students learn about the nursing process. This discussion has two sides. Decentralization allows decision-making closer to the patient and more autonomy at lower levels of an organization, but it can lead to variations in care from unit to unit and fragmentation of services. Consider how plans of care must ensure less decentralization and fragmentation to improve safety. Give students case scenarios, then discuss fragmented care, how it can be eliminated, and the role of the nurse in that effort. This can happen in clinical conferences, in the classroom, when students assess their patients, or when students discuss case studies. This does not require an additional lecture, only that the problem of fragmentation be identified and then woven into critical thinking activities and clinical experiences.

## Self-Management Support

Self-management support is "the systematic provision of education and supportive interventions to increase patients' skills and confidence in managing their health problems, including regular assessment of progress and problems, goal setting, and problem-solving support" (IOM, 2003b, p. 52). Self-management is particularly important in chronic illness, such as diabetes and asthma, and becomes even more complex when patients have multiple problems. Students need to consider self-management for every patient that they care for, and include the patient and the patient's family in the process.

### *Patient Errors in Self-Management*

Students need to understand that self-management allows patients to be more independent, but it also can lead to errors. How can patients be assisted in preventing these errors? Patients at risk include those with multiple chronic problems using multiple medications, and elderly patients trying to practice self-management in their homes. Teach students how to assist patients in using Medisets to administer their medication; how to monitor medication use by patients and caregivers; and how to teach patients and caregivers what to review when they receive their medications, such as drug name, dose, and so on. Give students a list of patient orders that include multiple oral medications with complex administration schedules, and ask them to prepare a Mediset based on these orders; they can fill the box with M&Ms in place of the pills. Put the medications in bottles with and without childproof lids and small print labels so they can appreciate that many factors (e.g., arthritis, poor eyesight) affect how a patient practices self-management. This simulation will help the student understand how easy it is for a patient to make an error. Are errors made in the simulation? What would be easy ways to make an error? How might this information be helpful in teaching patients and their families about Medisets? Use role playing, with students as the nurse, the patient, and family members. As they work through the simulation they learn better ways to educate patients, prevent errors, and help patients improve their own self-management.

## Healthcare Literacy

Healthcare literacy is "the ability to read, understand, and act on healthcare information" (IOM, 2003c, p. 52). It should be carefully considered in the development and use of teaching materials for patients and families. In particular, because students teach patients, students need to learn how to assess patient understanding and to make changes as required.

### *Self-Management and Health Literacy*

Students need to understand that self-management will not be effective if the patient has a low level of health literacy. Ask the student to explain why this would be. What skills does the patient need to manage his diabetes or her arthritis? Include health literacy problems in case examples related to adult health, pediatrics, mental health, obstetrics, or community health; it will help students to appreciate that health literacy issues can arise in all types of situations and can have an important impact on care and outcomes.

Students may have a difficult time appreciating what health literacy means and how it affects patient care. First, ask students to define health literacy. They may then need assistance imagining the shame and stigma that illiterate patients may experience. Role play may be useful here: provide students with information such as an admission form or patient education forms in a different language, then ask a student playing the role of the nurse to teach a patient, played by another student, about their disease and give the patient the written information. This could actually be in another language (most hospitals have this information at least in Spanish), which would give the student a more realistic experience. However, even using material in English can be a challenge, as many examples are not easily understood even by a native speaker. Afterwards discuss how the students felt and what the class observed. Have the students compare the definition of health literacy used in the IOM report with their own definitions. Ask them how the inability to read prescriptions or discharge instructions might be dangerous. In Spanish *once per day* translates to *una vez por día*. However, the English word *once* is spelled exactly like the Spanish word for *eleven*. So a Spanish speaker trying to read an English prescription could think that the patient needs the medication eleven times per day. This exercise also ties in with the IOM themes of quality of care and patient safety.

### *Interpreters*

If possible, students should work with an interpreter to facilitate communication with a patient. Students can experience the frustration of trying to communicate through a third party, and then discuss how it feels. They need guidance in using an interpreter; for example the student should talk directly to the patient not to the interpreter. This also is a good time to discuss the advantages and disadvantages of depending on family members to act as interpreters. What might be the impact of a different culture where the husband makes decisions: will the wife feel comfortable expressing herself, and will the husband try to soften difficult messages? Would it be better to use a native speaker or a language expert to interpret? Would distance from the patient ensure accurate translations instead of emotional ones? Discuss the options if there is no interpreter: finding a healthcare provider who speaks the language, working with community groups to help interpret, preparing visual materials that might aid communication, and so on.

### *Health Education and Health Literacy*

Give students consent forms, admission forms, and patient rights information, and let them assess their own ability to understand them. Ask them what might interfere with reading and understanding what they have read. What would help them understand the documents? Students have some healthcare background, but what about patients and families who have none? During clinical experiences, ask students how health literacy might affect teaching specific patients. This can also be done during pre- and postconferences.

### *The Healthcare Delivery System and Health Literacy*

What is done in a specific healthcare organization to address health literacy? How do health agencies used for clinical experiences respond to health literacy in their patient education programs? Students can gather information, observe, interview staff, and review written materials and other types of educational materials such as videos that might be shown to patients. Students can then discuss what they have learned, what could be improved, and how.

### *Health Literacy and Nursing Assessment and Interventions*

Students can assess a population group in their community or an agency and its patients for health literacy levels, problems, interventions that might have been taken and outcomes, and consider other types of interventions that might improve health literacy. Health literacy should be part of individual patient assessments. Is health literacy included in the assessments expected of students? How should this assessment be done? Is it part of healthcare organization standard assessment forms? Compare assessment forms from different healthcare organizations or different services within an organization.

## Patient Education

Patient education is a complex process: information about the process and experience with patient education is included in all nursing curricula. If a patient does not have enough information, this can affect care. Some areas that require patient education are identified in the IOM reports, such as tobacco, alcohol, high-fat foods, and firearm injury prevention. Nurses in community settings typically include all these topics in community education, but nurses in other settings also need to counsel patients about these issues.

Patient education must be culturally sensitive because the meanings of health, illness, and death are not the same everywhere. For some Muslim families this plane of life is just one level, and to resuscitate the patient back to this level is not as important as honoring the predestination of life events. The saving of locks of hair or pictures of Indian babies who are dying is not culturally accepted in all families; these mementos bind the child to this earthly world and do not allow the child to reach the next.

### *Family or Caregiver Roles*

Ask students how patients and families might become more involved in the development of safety standards, and why this is important. Explore initiatives to increase patient and family involvement, for example, the National Patient Safety Foundation (http://www.npsf.org); Agency for Healthcare Research and Quality (AHRQ) patient materials (http://www.ahrq.gov); the Institute for Safe Medication Practice (http://www.ismp.org); state patient materials; and the JCAHO Speak Up campaign (http://www.jcaho.org).

Staff also need to know how to approach patients and families when errors have occurred, so discussing this with students is important. They need to understand what an error can mean to a patient and family, and how they might feel: anger, distrust of staff, or abandonment. What might be the effect the next time the patient seeks care? Why is it important to ask patients more than just dates of past hospitalizations? A bad past experience can affect current treatment, so knowing more can be helpful. Ask students to put themselves in the place of the patient or family member to gain a better understanding of their responses and how nurses might help them cope. Naturally, there may be legal implications when errors occur, so students need to understand this aspect and to whom they should go for consultation.

### *Consumer Perspectives on Healthcare Needs*

Staying healthy, getting better, living with illness or disability, and coping with the end of life are topics of the *Quality Report* and are also important parts of nursing care. The consumer perspective may help students to remember these critical elements when working with patients and their families. Ask students to explore what each of the components of the quality framework really means in practice. Patients may be asked to talk with students about the implications of these perspectives in their own lives. What do they mean to a person with diabetes, mental illness, breast cancer, or a family with a newborn? These perspectives can help students working with individuals, families, or groups in a variety of healthcare settings and in the community.

### *Care Coordination*

Care coordination needs to be a topic in all courses and clinical experience from the very beginning of every nursing program, whether undergraduate or graduate. What is the role of the nurse? How can care coordination be improved? What is the integrator role that some nurses play? What can nurses do to improve interdisciplinary or interprofessional care coordination? It is vital to ask students specific questions about coordination in clinical settings to stimulate them to use critical thinking and consider the need for coordination. When students prepare care plans, they should be expected to address care coordination. When they take part in case studies and simulations they should be expected to respond to questions related to care coordination. A patient information system such as the Cerner partnership with the University of Kansas School of Nursing can be integrated with case studies to search for missing data, identify areas needing more assessment, and then actually develop the plan of care and its evaluation as if the student were in the healthcare setting. The advantages of such partnerships are that the students learn by doing—using actual healthcare environment systems, employing critical thinking skills, and integrating technology.

## *Work on Interdisciplinary Teams*

*Cooperate, collaborate, communicate, and integrate care in teams to ensure that care is continuous and reliable.* (IOM, 2003a, p. 4)

Interdisciplinary teams work collaboratively and collegially, not in parallel. Each health professional does not plan one aspect of care in isolation; instead, all team members work together to plan and implement care.

### An Environment of Learning, Not Blame

Build a learning environment that allows for learning from errors and near misses, not one of blame. Policy and standards need to be clear. Communication needs to be open. Survey students to find out how they view the learning environment. What do they think will happen if they make an error or if they report a near miss? Do they know the difference between the two? What is their attitude toward errors? What do they see happening related to safety in the healthcare organizations where they go for clinical experience? A school's Student Nurses Association could support a campaign for a safety culture.

### Training in Teams

Working with medicine, respiratory therapy, and any other group that might be involved in a Code allows team members to learn the perspective that each individual brings to the situation. Providing interdisciplinary simulated experiences, so that each professional learns their role in this type of high-stress, high-risk intervention helps when the real-life situation arises. Interprofessional schools might organize an annual safety fair for students and faculty. This can help highlight safety concerns, current evidence-based practice, and other related issues. Assign students from different healthcare professional schools to teams and ask them to create a poster or display on a facet of safety or quality. This provides an opportunity to work as a team to plan, research, and implement the project.

## A Culture of Safety

Creating and sustaining a culture of safety should include the following: (1) an understanding of its essential elements, (2) the barriers to creating the culture, (3) strategies to create the safety culture, and (4) evaluation of results or outcomes (IOM, 2004). Safety orientation is necessary to prepare staff and to maintain the knowledge of safety. Trust is a key issue when the staff are asked to report errors and near misses—what will be the reaction, and will staff be blamed? Nurses face a major hurdle in accepting this new type of safety culture, because "nurses are trained to believe that clinical perfection is an attainable goal" (Jones, 2002; cited in IOM, 2004, p. 298) and that "'good' nurses do not make errors" (Banister, Butt, & Hackel, 1996; cited in IOM, 2004, p. 298). Every nursing program needs to examine its culture periodically and dispel such unrealistic expectations.

### *Proactive Responses*

Faculty need to consider safety issues when changes are made in curriculum or in simulation labs, so that students know how to prevent errors in practice and how to respond to errors. Use scenarios that include errors to prompt students to demonstrate or at least explain what they would do if the error occurred, and discuss how teamwork would change the outcome. Set up the simulation lab with potential risks and errors, then ask students to identify them and recommend solutions.

## Safety Culture in the Healthcare Organization

Many HCOs are working to create safety cultures, and students are introduced to this in their practica. Students also should be told to ask about safety when they seek positions. Provide students with positive examples like the Veteran's Hospital Administration (VHA) system. Information is online at http://www.va.gov; the site describes the VHA safety culture, root cause analysis, and more. Ask students to search the Internet for other HCOs with information about safety on their web sites.

### *Stakeholders*

Many stakeholders are involved in the healthcare process, and it is important that students understand who the stakeholders are and what their roles are. Ask students how a patient is admitted to the hospital, and which stakeholders the patient will encounter. How does this affect quality of care, or fragmentation of care and care coordination, or the risk of errors?

### Change Process

Students should be familiar with the change process and be able to apply it in the clinical setting. Discuss change in pre- and postconferences; ask how change affects individual patients and their families, the patient care unit and its staff, and the healthcare organization, and how change affects the student. The faculty, however, needs to be a positive role model; demonstrate the ability to deal with constant flux instead of clinging to the status quo. Content needs to include redesigning care processes based on best practices; use of information technology; knowledge management; development of effective teams; coordination of care across patient conditions, services, and settings; performance and outcome measurements; organizational climate; and how to cope with change. Why are these issues important in health care; how do they affect nursing; and what related experiences have students had?

## *Need for Transparency*

Review how information is shared with patients or about patients, by whom, and what type of information. Include HIPAA implications. Why it is important for patients to be given information? As students participate in procedures they need to understand informed consent. They should be knowledgeable about organization policies and procedures. The best time to introduce informed consent and the nurse's role is when students learn about procedures.

### Teamwork

Every student needs both knowledge and experience working on teams. Schools of nursing typically include some of this content in their courses, but experience in teamwork is less common. Students can work in teams, but they need guidance and an opportunity to discuss the experience. They can be assigned to staff teams, and observe teams on a unit and then discuss their observations.

Team-based learning can be used in the classroom to teach students to apply knowledge as a team (Michaelsen, Knight, & Fink, 2004). First they complete an individual quiz on the content for the day, then they complete the same quiz with their team. The faculty review the answers with the teams, comparing responses and asking students for rationales for their responses. Cases are then used to assist the teams in applying the content. This method is now used in many colleges of medicine and some colleges of nursing.

### Nurses in Healthcare Organizations

Nurses are very involved in surveillance, which includes assessing or monitoring patients, delivering therapeutic interventions, and coordinating and integrating care from multiple providers (IOM, 2004). It is imperative that this role be communicated to nursing students and required of them. The nurse's role in HCOs is not static; consequently, nursing education needs to be aware of changing roles and modify what is taught. This, of course, must be correlated with current standards of practice. All of this requires that nursing education be able to make changes in curricula and teaching strategies in a more timely manner than today.

## Transformational Leadership

Transformational leadership is highly regarded today, and the IOM reports rate it as the best approach. This, however, does not mean that it is easy to implement; it is not. Students need to understand leadership and followership, and to appreciate how they respond as leaders and as followers. What makes an effective leader and an effective follower?

Most organizations are in a state of perpetual change; engage students in discussions of how they respond to change. They will soon have to step up, take a stand, be a leader, and this should begin while they are students. What is empowerment, and why is it important to nurses? Shared governance is one approach that has proven successful in developing a positive work climate. As students visit HCOs, faculty need to guide them in asking questions about leadership and organizational effectiveness. How does the organization respond to change? How well does the staff trust leadership? Why would this be important to know before taking a new position? Ask the students to consider the need for a close fit between their personal values and the values and mission of the organization. Ask about whistle blowing regulations and the implications if a student decides to be a real agent for change.

## Maximizing Workforce Capability

### *Promoting Safe Staffing Levels*

Patient safety and quality care are possible only if the problems of recruitment and retention are solved. Nursing students need assistance in job hunting skills such as interviewing, looking for a positive work environment, resumé and query letter writing, and finding a job that matches their competencies and personal needs. Schools of nursing could also reduce attrition by making clear to students what they may experience the first year, and cultivating skills like stress management, assertiveness, and problem solving.

### *Knowledge and Skill Acquisition*

Students experienced in working on a team, delegating, prioritizing, managing conflict, and critical thinking are more successful in their first jobs. Students also need experience recognizing when they need more information and where to find it, such as professional literature, the Internet, government resources, and experts. This recognizes that learning is a lifelong pursuit. Greater use of preceptors, especially near the end of a nursing program, can help students gain important competencies, confidence, and better understanding of professional roles and teamwork. Faculty need to be aware that some state regulations disallow substantial precepted hours in nursing programs, and that this can affect quality of education, patient safety, and the nursing shortage.

#### *Interdisciplinary Collaboration*

Precursors to collaboration are individual clinical competence and mutual trust and respect. Collaboration requires shared understanding of goals and roles, shared decision-making, and conflict management. Students need formal experience with collaboration so that they can receive support and guidance from faculty. They must learn how to have a respectful professional dialogue that considers many different perspectives. Students also need to understand how the history of nursing has fostered permissive, submissive language and actions (Gordon, 2005). See Appendix K for an example of an intraprofessional review of *Nursing Against the Odds*, a book that can be used to broaden the discussion to an interprofessional one.

#### *Verbal Abuse*

Communication skills are always important and should be developed throughout the curriculum; however, a growing concern for nurses is verbal abuse from other staff, physicians, and family members. In fact, verbal abuse is cited as one of the reasons that nursing is a stressful profession. Students need guidance in how to respond and examples of the strategies that some HCOs are using to prevent verbal abuse. Schools of nursing should also establish a policy of no tolerance of verbal abuse.

### Structured Interdisciplinary Forums

Structured interdisciplinary forums such as team planning, team rounds, meetings, and task groups are important opportunities to learn about collaboration, interdisciplinary issues, planning, communication, and how to work with others. They allow the student time to assess situations and learn from them with faculty support.

### Work and Work Space Design

#### *Design of Work Hours*

Students need information about fatigue and its effects on work: slowed reaction time, diminished attention to detail, errors of omission, compromised problem solving, reduced motivation and decreased vigor for successful completion of required tasks; the circadian rhythm; reactions to working a night shift and how shift work is arranged; adjusting to changing hours. Discuss how these factors affect the quality of care and the risk of errors to help students recognize the many factors that affect safe care. This can initially be done in the simulation lab and then re-emphasized during clinical experiences. Students need to be prepared for work, and should also learn how to prevent fatigue whenever possible. Mandatory overtime is a growing concern in health care today. What do students know about it? *Keeping Patients Safe* (IOM,

2004) recommends that nurses not work more than 12 hours in any 24-hour period or more than 60 hours in any seven-day period. If this occurs, it should be disclosed to the public. Students can research what their own states are doing about the problem at the ANA website (http://www.nursingworld.org), search nursing literature, and investigate working conditions in local HCOs.

### *Medications*

One of the interventions with the highest risk for error is medication administration, particularly given the increasing number of drugs, unfamiliarity with drugs, inadequate math proficiency, environmental stresses (interruptions, fatigue, overwork, and miscommunication), illegible orders, lack of patient information, and problems with equipment. Bar codes, unit dose dispensing, smart infusion pumps, reference resources, and drug training can all reduce errors. Administering medications safely is one of the critical competencies that any nursing student learns. Simulation practice can be very beneficial, and testing competency in a simulated experience allows students to learn without harming patients.

### *Transfers*

Patient transfers are considered high-risk for errors. Transfers can involve gaps in care, miscommunication, and duplication of effort. Interunit transfers have increased. "It is not unusual to see a patient cared for by five different nursing units during one hospital stay—for example, operating room, post-anesthesia care unit (PACU), critical care unit, step-down unit, and general medical-surgical unit—during his or her hospital stay" (IOM, 2004, p. 251). Students should consider why transfers increase the risk of errors. Ask them to brainstorm all the possible errors that might occur, and instill in them an awareness of the nurse's role during transfer and the need to consciously prevent errors. What could then be changed in processes to decrease risk?

### *Paperwork*

Clinical documentation and paperwork seem to only increase, and this excessive paperwork also plagues schools of nursing. Students typically spend much of their time on written assignments. It is difficult for faculty to step back and ask whether the assignments are helpful, whether they aid learning, meet course objectives, or develop competencies. What is the student perspective of the assignments? Requiring nursing students to write everything down may interfere with their ability to think on their feet, discuss an issue or problem, and use critical thinking. Some written assignments accomplish this, but not all. It is always difficult to give up a course activity after it has become routine, but if schools of nursing are to graduate competent entry-level nurses who can function in an ever-changing healthcare environment, nursing faculty too need to change and be willing to concede that a strategy or learning activity is not yielding expected outcomes.

### *Physical Plant*

Students probably do not think much about work space, but it is important. Ask students to assess a unit that they are on for practicum—describe the lighting, space, accessibility for patients, families, and staff, nurses' work area, noise, furnishings, traffic through the unit. What is their first impression when they step onto the unit? How does the unit atmosphere make them feel? For example, when Neonatal Intensive Care Units (NICUs) were traditional open rooms with no noise abatement, most of the nurses felt anxious and tense because of noise and bright lights. When more attention was paid to dimming lights and banning overhead pages, and more units were designed as pods or modules, staff became more careful to talk softly, more mindful of noise and lights, and less tense.

Ask students how the environment and work space affect how care is provided and received or increases the risk of errors. What could be changed to improve the work space? What could be done, that is not too costly and complex, to make the unit a better place to deliver and receive care? Students may have many creative ideas.

## Contingent Workers

HCOs are using more contingent workers (temporary agency nurses and traveling nurses) to fill empty positions. This costly solution affects employee morale and probably safety and quality of care. It is also a growing problem for nursing education. Contingent workers who work with students may not be fully aware of the HCO's policies, procedures, and communication systems or even willing to assist with teaching and supporting students. If a practicum requires the use of preceptors, it may be difficult to find enough qualified preceptors who are regular employees. It is important for faculty to know about the types of staff on units. Schools of nursing need to work with HCOs to determine how best to utilize available staff as effective preceptors, and how to prepare and support preceptors. If contingent nurses must be used for preceptors, and in some cases this cannot be avoided due to the shortage, then faculty, HCOs, and regulatory boards need to work together to make the experience safe and effective.

## Learning Organizations

The concept of learning organizations, in which the organization explicitly recognizes the importance of ongoing learning for its staff, is used in many Fortune 500 companies to stay abreast of changes and to encourage retention of staff. This same concept is now being used in HCOs and schools of nursing as the profession begins to recognize nurses as knowledge workers and knowledge as intellectual capital. Have students consider why it would be important to understand the learning organization and how it might affect patient safety. When students consider accepting a position, why should they consider the learning environment within the organization? Is learning an expectation in the HCO? Does the administration support lifelong learning either financially or with time off? Faculty can help students choose questions to find out if an HCO is a learning organization. What type of orientation is provided for new staff? Is there a mentorship or internship? If so how long does it last? What education is provided, by whom, for whom, and can staff get time off to attend education within the organization? Does the organization cover any education fees for academic courses or for continuing education courses? Is cross-training offered when the staff are expected to work in different areas? It is also important to find out how Unlicensed Assistive Personnel (UAPs) are trained and the type of additional training they receive. RNs may be expected to provide some training on the job, though this is not recommended. New graduates are not prepared for this role. Answers to these questions indicate how committed the organization is to staff education and to supporting a learning organization. Students could assess an HCO to determine whether it is a learning organization.

They should also ask about the organization's attitude toward knowledge and the sharing of information. Ask them to assess the educational programs offered by an HCO over a particular period. What types and content of programs were offered, and how often? Were they appropriate to the competencies required in the HCO? Does the schedule meet the needs of staff who work on different shifts? Are instructors qualified? How does the staff rate the quality of education? The goal is to get the students thinking about what is an effective learning environment. Magnet hospitals have high levels of training and education for their staff, and are more successful in recruitment and retention.

Students also need to explore their individual responsibility to improve competency. Lifelong learning is critical for any professional nurse today. Assigning students to attend a Continuing Education (CE) program and critique the program is another strategy to help students understand the need for lifelong learning. They can also explore the certification process in a specialty that interests them.

### Nurse Internships and Residencies

Nurse internships and residencies have been used in the past and are now increasing again. These programs help new graduates transition to practice, and offer a host of opportunities to expand their competencies. American Association of Colleges of Nursing (AACN) has partnered with some HCOs to pilot a standardized postbaccalaureate residency program, the first of which was implemented in 2002 (IOM, 2004). The results of this pilot are not yet available; however, the results will be important to nursing education and healthcare delivery. Many HCOs are also developing these programs themselves.

The concept is also part of the new role proposed by AACN: Clinical Nurse Leader (CNL). There is increasing funding for similar programs, like the Robert Wood Johnson (RWJ) Graduate Nursing and Medical Residents at the University of Rochester and Vanderbilt. The CNL role is aimed at the integration of services at the point of care by a nurse who is not a manager, not just a direct caregiver, but rather a person who coordinates services or case-manages the patient and family. At the University of Oklahoma Breast Institute a nurse navigator assists the patient and family through the complexity of screening, diagnosis, and management of any problems.

This role evolved out of the IOM reports and the emphasis on patient-focused, safe care. As these care models increase in number, it is important to see the new role a registered nurse and possibly a CNL will play. The necessary skills must be taught: critical thinking, resource management, and patient-focused care instead of serving the healthcare delivery system, and analysis of critical patient needs and how the interprofessional team provides comprehensive care.

## *Employ Evidence-Based Practice*

*Integrate best research with clinical expertise and patient values for optimum care, and participate in learning and research activities to the extent feasible.* (IOM, 2003a, p. 4)

"Evidence-based practice" means translating research findings into practice. Part of this discussion is to move the emphasis to evidence and how one levels or evaluates expert opinions and research findings instead of putting research first. Students are fearful of research, but they can embrace a scientific foundation for interventions and see the application in practice.

### Evidence-Based Practice

Sigma Theta Tau (2006) defines evidence-based practice (EBP) as "integration of best clinical practice, research evidence, nursing expertise, and the values and preferences of the individuals, families, and communities who are served" (http://www.nursingsociety.org). Some schools of nursing have changed their research courses to an evidence-based methodology, particularly for undergraduate students. In other courses, such as those with practica (e.g., pediatrics, adult health, mental health, family-focused, community) it is important that faculty incorporate evidence-based practice. The Academic Center of Evidence-Based Practice at the University of Texas Health Science Center in San Antonio has published *Essential Competencies for Evidence-Based Practice in Nursing* (Stevens, 2005), a useful guide to developing EBP competencies at the undergraduate, masters, and doctoral levels. Browsing the Cochrane Collaborative Library (http://www.cochrane.org/index0.htm) or the Joanna Briggs Institute (JBI) (http://www.joannabriggs.edu.au/about/home.php) for systematic reviews and a collection of EBP guidelines will show students the linkages between the science of nursing and the art of delivering care (research to practice). Another good resource is the AHRQ Guideline Clearinghouse (http://www.guideline.gov/).

Students learning to support intervention choices should review EBP resources such as http://www.ahrq.gov in all clinical courses. Students need to know about systematic reviews of multiple primary investigations, practice guidelines, and how to use computer-based clinical decision support systems. Evidence-based guidelines promote quality of care, and these should be incorporated in all courses. Students can review guidelines and consider how they might affect the care of minorities. AHRQ evidence-based practice centers are important resources for students and faculty. The nursing profession needs to be actively involved in the development of these EBP centers and the evidence-based process, and then ensure that nurses can access information relevant to nursing care, not just for physicians. Students need to be familiar with Sigma Theta Tau (http://www.nursingsociety.org) and the Academic Center for Evidence-Based Practice (http://www.acestar.uthscsa.edu). The thread of EBP belongs in all nursing curricula. JBI has a software program called the RAPid (Rapid Assessment Protocol Internet database) reviews which can be integrated into a research course or even a nursing core course to teach students to evaluate a research article. It is part of the Critical Appraisal Network of JBI (http://www.joannabriggs.edu.au/about/evidence_apprais_groups_map.php). This resource allows faculty and students to judge whether an article is strong evidence to support a certain intervention. This activity also helps tie together research, EBP, and best practices.

### Research

Nurses need to be involved in safety and quality research and to participate in evaluating how nursing care is connected to safety and quality. The reports recommend expansion of nursing research to increase nursing's understanding of patient safety's relationship to nursing care and the role of nurses. Some of these recommendations are the rationale for the new nursing role of the CNL recommended by AACN in its 2003 white paper. This role emphasizes leadership, delegation, care coordination, financial management, and knowledge of information systems. The CNL curriculum from the College of New Jersey includes:

- NURS 506 Theory and Research for Advanced Nursing Practice
- NURS 501 Perspectives in Advanced Nursing Practice
- NURS 504 Advanced Human Pathophysiology
- NURS 503 Pharmacology for Advanced Nursing Practice
- NURS 604 Research and Evidence-Based Nursing for Advanced Nursing Practice
- NURS 603 Individual, Family, and Community Systems
- NURS 633 Advanced Holistic Health Assessment
- NURS 685 Health Promotion for Individuals, Families, and Communities
- NURS (TBA) Nursing Management of Chronic and Complex Conditions
- NURS (TBA) Practicum in the CNL Role

This coursework combines traditional master's level courses with emphasis on theory and research, evidence-based nursing, holistic care, and health promotion in the community. The University of Florida College of Nursing has a CNL program, and its curriculum threads are:

- Critical thinking and decision-making
- Communication
- Ethics
- Human diversity and cultural competence

- Global health care
- Professional development in the CNL role
- Accountability
- Assessment
- Nursing technology and resource management
- Professional values, including social justice

This curriculum plan emphasizes ethics, cultural competence, accountability, technology and resource management, and social justice, all of which are supported by IOM.

In addition to curriculum changes, funding streams for HCOs are also influenced by IOM. As noted in the reports, AHRQ should fund research to evaluate how the current regulatory and legal systems (1) facilitate or inhibit the changes needed for the twenty-first century healthcare delivery system, and (2) can be modified to support healthcare professionals and organizations working to accomplish the six aims. This work has yet to be completed. Nursing should be involved in this process so that nursing input can be included; critical issues such as licensure and liability are involved in this recommendation. Multiple state compact licensure, which has been instituted in some states, is an example.

Any improvement in care requires data, analysis, and practical solutions. Increased clinical research, effectiveness studies, health services research, and outcomes studies are all needed. Nursing is collecting data, but much more needs to be done in this area (Lamb, Jennings, Mitchell, & Lang, 2004). Collecting data takes time and is expensive, so the process needs to be as efficient as possible. Data also must be collected systematically or their validity will be suspect. More research should examine the critical factors in quality, such as staffing, shift hours, workload, control over practice, collaboration, and communication.

Nursing education is very involved in research. Some schools of nursing are studying these critical quality issues, though more should, as nursing is directly involved in quality of care. One area that requires further exploration is how the education process affects student performance and thereby performance in the workplace.

Areas for nursing research related to safety and quality include:

- Fragmentation of care
- Errors and error prevention
- Safe medication administration
- Priority areas of care
- Impact of technology (medical and information)
- Implementing the five core competencies
- Prevention of patient falls
- Care coordination
- Teamwork (impact, implementation in education)

- Operating room and surgery procedures
- Emergency departments
- Management of diagnostic tests, screening, and information
- Intensive care units—adult, neonatal, pediatrics
- Care of frail elderly (falls, decubitus, etc.)

## *Apply Quality Improvement*

*Identify errors and hazards in care; understand and implement basic safety design principles, such as standardization and simplification; continually understand and measure quality of care in terms of structure, process, and outcomes in relation to patient and community needs; and design and test interventions to change processes and systems of care, with the objective of improving quality.* (IOM, 2003a, p. 4)

This strategy focuses on quality improvement and adding checks and balances to the system to ensure continuous quality. This has been brought to the forefront by concern for patient safety and the role of medication errors.

### Errors

#### *Analysis*

When near misses or errors occur in practicum, ask the student to identify the type of error and to provide a rationale. Let the student discuss their reaction and feelings. Discuss possible steps to prevent the error. In a root cause analysis, look at system processes, considering teaching methods, learning opportunities, inexperienced faculty, or other factors that contributed to the error. Give students scenarios to analyze and determine which errors may lead to harm, and what type of harm. When students review scenarios, it is easy to jump to the conclusion that there was not enough staff; encourage them to look for many possible causes for an error.

#### *Simplistic Solutions*

In scenarios of safety problems, ask students for a variety of possible solutions. Give teams the same scenario, such as a medication error, then have the teams share their solutions to demonstrate the range of possible solutions.

#### *Human Factors*

Help students analyze errors and identify human factors that may be related to the errors, while reminding them that human factors are not always the cause. Analyze the event, causes, circumstances, conditions, associated procedures, and devices that may be involved. Students need to understand this process well enough to use it in their clinical practice. Discuss the effects of stressors on error rates, including job dissatisfaction, burnout, work overload, shift work, family issues, and organizational politics.

### *Legal Issues*

Include specific examples of legal issues, standards of practice, nurse practice acts, and documentation of errors.

## JCAHO and QI

### *JCAHO Accreditation*

Students need to understand the purpose of JCAHO accreditation and the basic elements of the process. If a local HCO is undergoing accreditation and students are in the organization for practicum, discuss what they can expect during the accreditation visit. Students may be able to attend some of the planning meetings. Invite a staff member involved in the accreditation planning to talk about the process and the plan. This is more important today because accreditors are spending more time with staff nurses.

### *Changes in JCAHO Standards*

Include JCAHO safety information in course content; for example, under documentation include abbreviations that should not be used. Even after students have completed documentation, they need to be informed of changes, to emphasize that even in practice they need to keep up with current safety and documentation requirements. The faculty will need to stay aware of the changes, so schools of nursing will need to ensure that this review is completed annually. This does mean that someone has to be assigned to check for updates, and perhaps post them to a convenient web site. Other updates related to standards, guidelines (AHRQ), safety and QI issues, EBP, FDA drug alerts (http://www.fda.gov), updates on nursing workforce safety (http://www.nursingworld.org), the annual National Quality report, and the annual Healthcare Disparity report can also be noted to give faculty easy access to current information.

## Medications and Administration: Errors

### *Increased Use of Drugs*

With more patients taking prescription, over-the-counter, and complementary medications, errors have increased. Students need to learn all the steps of medication administration, multiple drug use, patient and caregiver education and direction, how to question conflicting orders, and assessment of patient medication.

### *Use of Multiple Drugs*

Use simulation scenarios that include multiple drug orders for students to identify appropriate orders, drug interactions, dosage, and administration. Discuss typical errors or ask students what they think would be typical errors based on an analysis of the medication procedure. Ask what corrective actions they would take and what might prevent a future error.

### *Medication Process*

Each step in the medication process—prescribing, dispensing, administering, monitoring, and management—should be included in content and applied to practice. Begin when students first learn about medication administration, and reinforce it throughout the curriculum. Name confusion is a common cause of drug errors; provide examples and ask students to distinguish between them. The FDA is compiling standards to prevent name mix-ups and to avoid confusing packaging (Jones, 2001). See also JCAHO recommendations related to medication administration and documentation on their web site (http://www.jcaho.org). Inform students about the process for reporting medication errors within the HCO. There is also a system through the U.S. Pharmacopeia (USP) for reporting errors. The Institute for Safe Medication Practices (ISMP) includes cases and warnings on its web site (http://www.ismp.org). In legal and ethical course content, discuss malpractice and professional liability insurance.

### *Preventable Causes of Adverse Drug Events*

Methods such as the cause-and-effect diagram can help students explore preventable adverse drug events. Use these methods in simulations to analyze causes. Provide students with case studies and have them work in teams to develop a cause-and-effect diagram. Possible events include medication error, patient fall, wrong patient receiving a treatment, wound infection, and so on. This approach can help students to understand the implications of processes on care and outcomes.

### *New Approaches to Medication Administration*

Burnes-Bolton has initiated a new approach to medication administration at Cedar Sinai of Los Angeles. It blends the old and new in a collaborative approach to reduce medication errors. It poses four questions (Steefel, 2002): (1) What if an RN with advanced knowledge and experience worked in collaboration with pharmacy and medical staff to codesign the medication process? (2) What if an RN interviewed all newly admitted patients and set a medication plan? (3) What if an RN and a pharmacist co-led the patient or family education process at the unit or clinic level? (4) What if nurses applied the sterile cockpit process (no interruptions in the cockpit—in the case of nursing, no interruptions as medications are prepared and administered) to the medication administration process? These strategies and others will be explored in many hospitals to combat medication errors. Make students aware of these new approaches and ask them to consider different methods to improve the medication process with critical thinking. As RNs they will not have time to wait for others to come up with solutions.

## Effective Medication Management

In 2003, the list of priority areas for national action particularly labeled preventing medication errors and overprescription of antibiotics as critical concerns.

Pharmacology courses should explain the purpose of antibiotics, the risk of overprescription, and the results of overprescription. Nurses provide patient and family education in schools, clinics, hospitals, and many other settings where it is easy to incorporate information about appropriate use of antibiotics, especially in pediatrics. Ask students to list the antibiotics they have taken and for what reasons, to highlight the frequency of antibiotic prescriptions, which may not always be appropriate. What are the consequences for individuals and communities when antibiotics are used inappropriately?

### Safety in the Plan of Care

Clearly note where students should include information about safety in the care plans that they develop. If a standard template is used, include safety in the template to remind students to address it for every patient, as well as to recognize how safety needs may change for a patient.

### Wrong-Site Surgery Errors

The ANA has joined more than 40 organizations to endorse the use of a new Universal Protocol, which includes marking the surgical site, involving the patient in the marking process, and taking a final "time out" in the operating room to recheck with the entire team. This protocol refers to "Wrong-Site Surgery Errors." This content should be included in clinical content and practica when surgical patients are assigned to students. In simulation lab, students can demonstrate this protocol through role playing.

### Patient Falls

Patient falls are a safety concern for all nurses. The ANA National Database of Nursing Quality Indicators (NDNQI) (http://www.nursingquality.org/faq.htm) reports that falls continue to be a problem, occurring on all types of units, and that approximately 30% involved injury (Dunton, et al., 2004). Content should cover falls, risk assessment including history of falls, medication use and effects, decreased mental status, decreased mobility, physiological effects of aging, external environmental factors (Ignatavicius, 2000), and preventive interventions. Variations in patient populations should be noted in appropriate courses: elderly, children, postsurgery, and so on. This assessment should also be part of the safety element in care plans. This is also a good time to introduce the use of restraints and related safety interventions.

### Setting Safety Standards

Each school of nursing should set a minimum standard of safety for students. Safety standards established by nursing professional organizations should be incorporated into the curriculum; for example, standards in care of children should be included in pediatric content. Schools of nursing need to be aware of changes in FDA standards for medical products and monitoring their safety, in order to incorporate these into content and practicum. Students and faculty must also follow standards set by healthcare organizations where students obtain clinical experience. ANA publishes information about workplace safety that is important for students (http://www.nurisngworld.org).

### Infectious Diseases

Surveillance, prevention, and control of infectious diseases can be introduced when students begin to learn clinical competencies in simulated experiences, included in didactic content, and reinforced in the clinical setting. Let nursing staff who provide infection control services teach students. Students need to know and follow the infection control policies and procedures in organizations where they receive clinical experience. Postoperative infections have the most serious consequences of all medical injuries—increasing length of stay, treatment costs, and risk of death. Handwashing is critical and needs to be reinforced with students in simulation lab and in clinical. (See CDC Handwashing Guidelines at http://www.cdc.gov/handhygiene.) JCAHO also emphasizes handwashing in its surveys. In simulations, they should be asked what they would assess; in practica they should identify risks for acquiring and transmitting infectious agents. Students must use handwashing appropriately in all simulated experiences in order to make this a habit in clinical practice. Monitoring patients is a critical element of nursing that can reduce errors, and should be built into all nursing experiences. Ask students what and when they should monitor. What do monitoring results mean? What interventions should then be taken?

### Surgical Morbidity and Mortality Conferences, Autopsy

Morbidity and mortality (M&M) are common concepts in health care, and students need to understand how the healthcare organization analyzes M&M and uses the data. M&M are typically introduced in community health content, but are also relevant to acute care. AHRQ has created WebM&M with the University of California at San Francisco as a national forum to discuss and learn from medical errors (http://www.webmm.ahrq.gov). This site, which also provides power point slides of its cases, which change monthly, can be used to explore the problem of medical errors. Students will experience patients who die, so they need to understand how autopsy is used to improve care and reduce errors. Open discussion of this topic is essential.

### Risk Management

Risk management is a large program in most healthcare organizations. Students need to know its purpose and how it relates to patient care. This material may be included in management content. If a student makes an error in the clinical setting, the organization's incident report—some schools of nursing also have an incident report form—must be completed. This is a good time to reinforce risk management.

### Access to Care Management Programs and Guidelines

Students need to know what care management programs and clinical guidelines are and where to find them (also patient care protocols, clinical pathways, algorithms, and so on). These are particularly relevant for patients with chronic problems. How do these programs and guidelines apply to nursing care? Provide students with examples, which can be found on the Internet, and discuss the implications for nursing. Ask students to identify relevant programs and guidelines for their assigned patients and how they might use them in providing nursing care.

### Safety as a Competency

Because healthcare organizations need to review their competency requirements for new staff and to update staff over time about safety, schools of nursing need to also ensure that safety is included in their student competencies. These competencies should be consistent with staff competencies established by healthcare organizations. Schools of nursing should use local healthcare organizations' safety requirements and competencies, nursing professional standards, regulations (nurse practice acts), and JCAHO safety standards or those of other accreditation organizations.

### High-Risk Areas

The report on priority areas (IOM, 2003b) lists some critical high-risk areas that should be included in content and discussions with students. These are also potential research concerns for nursing. They include:

- Widely varied interactions with diagnostic or treatment technology; use of many different types of equipment,
- Multiple staff involved in the care of individual patients, and many hand-offs of care,
- High acuity of patient illness or injury,
- Environment prone to distractions or interruptions,
- Need for rapid decisions; caregivers being time-pressured,
- High-volume or unpredictable patient flow,
- Use of diagnostic or therapeutic interventions with a narrow margin of safety, including high-risk drugs,
- Communication barriers with patients or coworkers, and
- Instructional setting for care delivery, with inexperienced caregivers (IOM, 2004, p. 129).

### Six Aims

The six aims of quality care are safe, effective, patient-centered, timely, efficient, and equitable care. Each one of these is highly relevant to nursing. Ask students to determine how each one of the aims affects their assigned patient; how they affect an aggregate or population; what can be done to resolve problems that may block meeting these aims. Case studies, discussion, and clinical experience will make the student more aware of the aims and how they impact care. The aims may conflict at times, and it is important for students to discuss how this may occur and how it can be resolved. Can safe care always be efficient? Some of this discussion will involve ethics and legal issues.

### Clinical Content and Experiences

The following are specifically mentioned as important elements of content and clinical experience (IOM, 2001a, p. 209):

- Use a variety of approaches to deliver care, including the provision of care without face-to-face contact.
- Synthesize evidence and communicate it to patients.
- Combine evidence, knowledge about population outcomes, and patient preferences to individualize care.
- Communicate with patients openly to assist them in making decisions and self-management.
- Use decision support systems and other tools to assist in making decisions to reduce overuse, underuse, waste, and redundancy.
- Identify errors and hazards in care, and understand and implement basic safety design principles.
- Understand the course of illness and the patient's needs and experiences at home (the most critical training need).
- Continually measure quality of care (process and outcomes) and implement best practices.
- Work collaboratively in teams.
- Design processes of care and measure their effectiveness.
- Understand how knowledge continually changes and expands.
- Understand determinants of health, the link between medical care and healthy populations, and professional responsibilities.

Faculty need to ask how this content is currently taught and if not, how it could be included. Learning activities should be creative to encourage students to incorporate the ideas and content into their practice.

### National Healthcare Quality Report Matrix

Use this matrix to analyze cases and discuss patient care. Ask students to identify critical issues related to matrix components. Some may apply and some may not, depending on the case or the healthcare setting. The matrix is reproduced in Appendix D. The annual report is online at http://www.ahrq.gov/qual/nhqr03/nhqrsum03.htm.

### Priority Areas for National Action

The priority areas are patient services that consume much of the cost, staff resources, and so on. Schools of nursing need to include each priority area in curricula.

### *Care Coordination*

Clinical integration is defined as "the extent to which patient care services are coordinated across people, functions, activities, and sites over time so as to maximize the value of services delivered to patients" (Shortell, Gillies, & Anderson, 2000; as cited in IOM, 2003a, p. 49). Care coordination is an important aspect of all care. Students at all levels need to understand care coordination and describe the role of nursing. In clinical, ask students how care coordination could be improved, and have them participate in coordination in acute care and in the community. Several reports indicate that interdisciplinary care is important and needs to improve. Preparing nursing students to participate as members of interdisciplinary teams is a challenge. It will take time to build relationships with other healthcare faculty so that students get interdisciplinary experience. Schools of nursing that work toward this goal will excel, and their graduates will be better prepared to practice in the real world.

### *Adequate Pain Control*

Pain management is part of curricula in a variety of nursing courses. Most schools include more than just the use of medications to control pain, and have expanded into alternative pain control methods. Evidence-based practice becomes important as students learn about the varying effectiveness of methods in different patient populations. Students need opportunities to observe or use these alternatives. Spend extra time on pain control for cancer patients, and cover this when cancer is presented. Pain assessment is now referred to as the fifth vital sign, and JCAHO requires an assessment of pain; students need to understand why.

### *Asthma*

Asthma is an important subject for nursing students. Asthma affects all age groups in all settings. As in some other priority areas, students can assess the incidence of asthma in the community, compare these data with state and national data, investigate causes of asthma and types of treatment and their efficacy, and devise strategies for self-management. Disease management programs for asthma are available. What do students know about disease management programs? Why have these programs improved outcomes? What is the role of nurses in these programs? Preparing and delivering education to the community is also a helpful learning activity. Be sure students appreciate the importance of improved patient outcomes, understand the process, and consider the role of the nurse in improving care.

### *Obesity*

Obesity is a complex challenge. Include in discussion risk factors, prevention, nutrition, exercise, complications, pharmacology, and effects of drugs on weight, pathophysiology, and treatment and efficacy. Given its importance today, obesity needs to be discussed in many content areas: nutrition, pediatrics, pregnancy, adults, community, and mental health.

### *Major Depression*

Depression is typically taught in mental health courses. Content should keep pace with new developments including genetics and the questionable use of antidepressants with children. Depression affects people in all age groups and all settings. Students may assume that they will only encounter patients with depression in their mental health rotation, but faculty need to point out that it strikes other patients, for example, cancer patients, victims of myocardial infarction, postpartum mothers, and children. Students with clinical experience in public schools can explore the level of depression and suicide in various age groups. What type of education (e.g., self-esteem, depression, coping skills, suicide) do public school students need? At what age? In any setting, students need to understand that assessing depression should be part of a general assessment, not just something that is assessed in behavioral healthcare units or mental health clinics.

### *Nosocomial Infections*

The risk of nosocomial infections is high today. When students are first introduced to handwashing and to sterile technique they need be told about nosocomial infections—causes, prevention, and the role of nurses as well as the importance of reducing these infections to improve care. What is the impact of increased nosocomial infections on healthcare delivery—economic, quality of care, complications, and prolonged hospital stays?

### *Pregnancy and Childbirth*

Pregnancy and childbirth are normally positive, healthy experiences, but when they are not, it affects the mother, the newborn, and family members. Preventing complications and adverse outcomes is a critical goal. Tobacco cessation, another priority area, should be part of care for all pregnant women. There are also serious racial and ethnic disparities. Students can explore these issues within their community and then apply the information to their experiences in clinical settings.

### *Severe and Persistent Mental Illness*

Severe and persistent mental illness is not an easy topic for students. They may experience a sense of hopelessness. Students do need to understand serious mental illness, its impact on the patient, family, and community, types of treatment and their efficacy and side effects, and outcomes to improve care. When students investigate the types of treatment and support services available in the community, it is usually an eye opener. Discuss the issue of parity and the current status of legislation at the state and national levels.

This topic typically involves ethical and legal issues. Do staff have the right to force medications on patients? What patient rights are important and how are they protected? What is involved in commitment? Why should this "chronic" illness be any different than diabetes or some other chronic illness? Providing some clinical experience with this population is important; students will encounter patients with severe and persistent mental illness in all settings, because such patients do experience other types of medical problems.

### *Stroke*

Stroke is covered in nursing curricula, and typically includes the full range of content and settings where patients receive treatment, from emergency room to rehabilitation and home. All curricula should do more in discussing quality of life and disabilities.

### *Tobacco Dependence*

Tobacco dependence is the "single most preventable cause of disease and death" (IOM, 2003b, p. 89). Students need information about risks, prevention, age groups and why each group might require different strategies to decrease dependence, the dependence process, complications, and methods used to help individuals stop smoking. Students need to also understand the impact of politics and economics on the availability of tobacco.

### *Cancer Screening*

Cancer screening should be evidence-based. The focus at this time is on colorectal and cervical cancer. Students can be provided information about the screening for these two types of cancer as well as observe a screening program. Students can research the rates of colorectal cancer and cervical cancer in their local community. How does it compare with the state and the nation? What screening is being done and by whom? What are the outcomes of the screening efforts? What could be done to improve the outcomes?

### *Children with Special Needs*

Some schools of nursing offer content or specific courses on the care of children with special needs. Students often encounter children with special needs during clinical experiences in schools or in acute care pediatric settings. These children have complex needs—physical, emotional, family, financial, and so on. Care coordination is an important part of the care for this population. What are the community resources for children with special needs? Are they easy for families to access? What type of help do caregivers need?

### *Diabetes*

Diabetes is a growing problem and is an important content area for nursing students. Diabetes affects patients in all age groups and all settings. Working with diabetic nurse educators or in a diabetic clinic is a helpful learning experience. Involvement with the local chapter of the American Diabetic Association will help students understand the role of consumers in self-advocacy, and the resources available in the community.

### *End of Life*

Today practice centers on congestive heart failure and obstructive pulmonary disease. More and more information is now available for schools of nursing about end-of–life (EOL) issues. The Hartford Foundation (http://www.hartfordign.org) offers important information that can enhance content and student experiences. Many schools of nursing are also participating in the AACN End-of-Life-Nursing Education Consortium (ELNEC), which is furthering the task of integrating EOL and palliative care into nursing curricula and teach-the-teachers for continuing education. Hospitals and healthcare facilities are forming palliative care teams in response to patients who want to be allowed to die a natural death and to be provided adequate pain control. These are skills that student nurses need to provide comforting care and anticipate family and patient needs in the face of a life-threatening or terminal illness.

### *Frailty Associated with Old Age*

Preventing falls and pressure ulcers, maximizing function, and developing advanced care plans are all key nursing concerns. Information about aging and the needs of the aged population is online at the Hartford Foundation (http://www.hartfordign.org). What type of clinical experience do students have with this population? Many students do not like working with the elderly; however, it is important clinical experience, given the aging of the population. Faculty should examine their own attitude toward this patient population and toward nurses who work in this specialty; it may not be positive, and they may be sharing it with students, perhaps unconsciously.

Begin by emphasizing fall prevention throughout the curriculum. Ask students to evaluate their patients' fall risk and skin condition, which must be part of routine care. Healthcare organizations are emphasizing this with their staff, and JCAHO is also including it as an important part of their standards and accreditation surveys. How do students plan to maximize patient function? Students need to be specific and consider individual needs and limitations. Preventing falls and pressure ulcers, and maximizing function, are also potential fields for nursing research. Some has been done but more is needed because nursing care can influence outcomes.

Advanced care plans need to be understood. Students need an opportunity to consider these complex needs and how they feel about them. The goal is "to provide integrated dignified care for those of advanced age" (IOM, 2003b, p. 47). Students need to provide care that is respectful of patient and family wishes, and this is not always easy. It is best to work through these issues while a student. Pre- and post-conference are good places to address them.

### *Hypertension*

Care for hypertension mostly means management of early disease before it becomes worse. Hypertension is typically included in content. Students, however, also need to understand the need for prevention, early detection, and strategies to help newly diagnosed patients. What screening is done in the community and by whom? Students may participate in screenings. Ask students what could happen if a person is not diagnosed early.

### *Immunization*

Immunization is important to children and adults. Each year awareness campaigns remind people about the need for immunization. Often nursing students participate in community immunization clinics or drives. While the United States has done better in recent years to get children immunized, the reality is that continued immunization of adults for diphtheria, pertussis, and tetanus (DPT) has not kept up. Fear of terroristic use of infectious agents, and the spread of global infections such as Avian Flu and SARS, have revealed the vulnerability of adults to common illnesses. Have students research the outbreaks of infectious agents for which immunizations are available and correlate them with vulnerable age groups who should received immunizations. Students can search the Internet for information about national and state efforts to improve immunization rates and compare them with local efforts. (See http://www.cdc.gov for updates on immunization requirements.)

### *Ischemic Heart Disease*

Ischemic heart disease is the leading cause of death for men and women. The critical elements of prevention, reduction of recurring events, and optimization of functional capacity should be included in content related to ischemic heart disease. Students should also be asked to explain how these apply to their patients.

## Framework for Building Patient Safety

Schools of nursing can use the framework for building patient safety to create a learning environment that engenders patient safety. The framework dictates the adoption of safeguards against foreseeable hazards. The following are some of the defenses that nursing education might employ:

- Student safety and quality care competencies incorporated into student evaluation
- Quality of faculty teaching and clinical expertise
- Creating and maintaining a blame-free culture
- Clear communication among faculty and students about courses and learning experiences
- Consistent course content and expectations
- Faculty teamwork and planning
- Up-to-date curriculum (evidence-based practice, IOM reports, AHRQ material, and so on)
- Evaluation of competency that includes patient safety concerns
- Supportive faculty willing to work with students
- Knowledge of clinical setting (staffing and qualifications of staff, policies and procedures, culture related to safety, environmental risks that increase errors)

### Occupational Health

Mention the Occupational Safety and Health Administration (OSHA) and the National Institute for Occupational Safety and Health (NIOSH) when discussing the health needs of employees. Students can access the web sites (http://www.OSHA.gov and http://www.NIOSH.gov) to learn more. How do the agencies relate to employers and employees? Some nursing programs use occupational health settings for practica and explore the role of the occupational health nurse. Students can participate in screening efforts and health education programs that might be offered in the work setting. Students can explore the health risks for specific work settings and strategies used to prevent problems in each. Students should understand worker's compensation and how it differs from private and other government forms of health insurance. They should also be asked to list the companies in their area that have dropped health insurance for employees or cut back their contribution to coverage, and evaluate the impact on vulnerability of the population to disease. Students should consider the number of uninsured and underinsured in their state. Then they can compare the percentage of gross national product spent on health care in the United States to other countries with better morbidity and mortality rates for childbearing women and children in particular.

## *Utilize Informatics*

*Communicate, manage knowledge, mitigate error, and support decision-making using information technology.* (IOM, 2003a, p. 4)

Use of informatics emphasizes the need to use data collected by HCOs to manage patient information, protect the patient against errors, and support healthcare interventions. Data mining is a common practice in business, but has only recently been effectively used in health care.

Technology is an asset in today's healthcare delivery system, but it can also be problematic. Technology is not only used in providing care, it has also become a widely recommended tool to decrease errors. Locsin (2005) comments that with the increasing use of medical technology there is concern about nurses losing the caring aspects of nursing. Help students understand the major contributions of technology to health care, but also discuss the implications for how care is provided and the impact it may have on the nurse–patient relationship. How can the "care" be kept in nursing care in a critical care unit that is so dependent on medical technology?

There is a perception that technology will lead to fewer errors than strategies that focus on staff performance; however, technology may in some circumstances lead to more errors. This is particularly true when the technology fails to take into account the end users, increases staff time, replicates an already bad process, or is implemented with insufficient training. The best approach is not always clear, and most approaches have advantages and disadvantages. We need to learn how to make technology safer, and when to rely on people instead. According to AHRQ, technology can be effective in providing computerized monitoring of adverse drug events, computer-generated reminders for follow-up testing, computerized POEs (this terminology implies an emphasis on physicians and is changing to *electronic health record* and *professional order entry* to recognize an interprofessional effort to automate documentation), automated dispensing of medication, handheld devices for prescription information, electronic health records that can provide portable birth-to-death data, and online support groups for patients (AHRQ, 2003). In addition, AHRQ recognizes the need to develop information technology standards in health care and will lead this effort.

### Use of Computers in Healthcare Organizations

Students need experience working with computers in healthcare settings. Though not all healthcare organizations will use the same software, understanding the principles of computerized documentation systems is critical. Identifying common errors is helpful. There is a need to make technology competencies critical skills and terminal objectives of our educational programs. Students need to know how the Health Insurance Portability and Accountability Act (HIPAA) applies to computerized systems. The Safety Report emphasizes the need for shared knowledge and the free flow of information—it needs to be "interactive, real-time, and prospective" (IOM, 2001a, p. 72). This requires effective use of information technology, and students need to begin learning about it in school.

### Computer-Based Reminder Systems

Students need to understand how these systems work and how they may assist nurses, for example, reminding nurses of risks for patient falls, allergies, and times for medication or specific monitoring. If local healthcare organizations include this type of support in their information technology, students can appreciate how this information can help them provide better care.

### Access to Complete Patient Information at the Point of Care

What is the value to nursing care of access to patient information at the point of care? Encouraging students to consider this will help them to understand how they can use the information and how this can eliminate errors and near misses.

### Clinical Decision Support Systems

With today's expanding and rapidly changing knowledge, nurses have a difficult time keeping current. Building this knowledge into information technology to help nurses make better decisions should be just as important as doing this for physicians. Students and faculty have installed pharmacology information in their personal digital assistants (PDAs), and this is one example of how technologies can help in decision-making. Faculty can instruct students in the most effective usage of these tools.

### HIPAA

The new information infrastructure must meet HIPAA requirements. Show students how HIPAA requirements apply to their practice, as students as well as after graduation. Schools of nursing are already very involved in ensuring that HIPAA requirements are met, but these requirements can easily be forgotten, so students need reminders (as do faculty).

## *Summary*

Many strategies could be used to respond to the IOM concerns and recommendations. We have described some strategies that can be tried. Hopefully they will stimulate faculty to be creative in their teaching, and encourage greater use of the valuable information and recommendations found in the IOM reports.

# Part 4

# Using IOM Reports in the Classroom

Part 4 contains examples that nursing faculty can use to incorporate content and recommendations from the IOM reports. The following are the areas covered in these teaching strategies for the classroom and clinical experiences. The companion CD-ROM includes additional strategies.

- Learning Objectives
- Presentations
- Teaching tips and techniques
- Issues for further exploration
  - Current events
  - Fields of study
  - Cross-cultural education
  - Future implications
- Classroom activities—this section includes:
  - Story sharing
  - A case study
  - Root cause analysis
  - Steps in critical thinking
  - Discussion questions and essay questions
- Self-assessment tools
- Questions for reflection
- Test questions (including a sample test with answers)

## *Learning Objectives*

The student will be able to:

1. Describe the major IOM reports on quality, safety, and diversity.
2. Discuss the nursing implications of these IOM reports.

3. Recognize how the nursing profession is responding to safety and quality concerns in healthcare delivery and as part of an interprofessional team.
4. Explain how the five healthcare professions core competencies apply to the student's learning and consequent practice.

## *Presentations*

The CD-ROM contains PowerPoint slides for the following presentations: (1) Healthcare Safety, (2) Healthcare Quality, (3) Public Health: Safety and Quality, (4) Healthcare Diversity, and (5) Evidence-Based Practice. The presentations include slides, objectives, relevant notes, Internet resources, and teaching strategies. In addition there is a commentary on the book *Nursing Against the Odds* by Suzanne Gordon. Use such books in classroom discussions to illustrate interprofessional learning and to model respectful dialogues.

## *Teaching Tips and Techniques*

Previous sections list many ways that the IOM's directives and recommendations can be used in teaching. Examples of curricular plans for CNL and DNP programs have been described in Parts 2 and 3. This section gives several examples of presentations to be used and adapted for teaching. In addition other strategies include:

- Create blogs (personal web sites that others can add comments to but not alter) for discussion of topics such as patient safety.
- Create wikis (web sites that allow multiple authors to comment and edit documents or the site itself) for discussion.
- Conduct threaded discussions in online classrooms.
- Assign students to search the Internet for instances of these concepts in healthcare delivery and health professional education.
- Investigate computerized medical records or physician order entry systems to find out what types of information are integrated, who has access, and how they comply with HIPAA.
- Select an error that has occurred either in a patient care setting or in a school of nursing and have the students conduct a root cause analysis.
- Apply the principle of patient-centered care to a clinical scenario where a student is the patient. Base all decisions in care on the patient's point of view: schedule of treatments, medications, what treatments to have, and what to refuse. Then discuss how that differs from traditional care.
- Ask students to either find or create examples of continuous quality improvement in healthcare delivery and schools of nursing. Discuss how well they work. If they find no such systems in educational programs, ask why not.

- Have graduate students describe how care delivery has changed since they completed their undergraduate studies. Have them describe what, if any, impact the IOM reports have had.
- Have graduate or undergraduate students discuss the rationale behind the movement to create BSN-MPH and MD-MPH or PhD in public health dual degrees.

## *Issues for Further Exploration*

The IOM reports are just beginning to change nursing education. Further speculation or anticipation of needed changes in our educational systems may be beneficial.

### Current Events

Current events that are relevant to the IOM reports include:

- Outbreaks of avian flu
- Outbreaks of SARS
- Ineffective response to natural disasters such as the 2004 tsunami, hurricanes, and earthquakes
- Concerns over healthcare costs and quality of care

### Fields of Study

Among the topics that IOM is studying, some that affect nursing and healthcare delivery are:

- Aging
  - Evidence-Base Medicine Roundtable
  - Disability in America
  - Health Insurance Is a Family Matter
  - Improving the Quality of Long-Term Care
  - Approaching Death: Improving Care at the End of Life
  - Disability in America: Toward a National Agenda for Prevention
- Diseases
  - The Economics of Antimalarials
  - Smallpox Vaccination Program Implementation
  - Shortening the Time Line for New Cancer Treatments
  - Saving Women's Lives: Strategies for Improving Breast Cancer Diagnosis
  - Evidence-Based Medicine Roundtable
  - Public Financing and Delivery of HIV Care
  - Cancer Survivorship: Improving Care and Quality of Life
- Education
  - The Future of Emergency Care in the United States Health System

    - Roundtable on Health Literacy
    - Nutritional Standards for Foods in Schools
    - Educating Public Health Professionals for the Twenty-First Century
    - Assessing Integrity in Research Environments
- Public Health
    - Workshop on Estimating the Contribution of Lifestyle-Related Factors to Preventable Death
    - Progress in Preventing Childhood Obesity
    - Genomics and the Public's Health in the Twenty-First Century
- Child Health
    - Review of the National Immunization Program's Research Procedures and Data Sharing Program
    - Postmarket Surveillance of Pediatric Medical devices
    - Developing a Strategy to Reduce and Prevent Underage Drinking
- Food and Nutrition
    - Framework for Evaluating the Safety of Dietary Supplements
    - Safety of Genetically Engineered Foods: Approaches to Assessing Unintended Health Effects
- Mental Health
    - Gulf War and Health: Physiologic, Psychologic, and Psychosocial Effects of Deployment-Related Stress
    - Crossing the Quality Chasm: Adaptation to Mental Health and Addictive Disorders
- Military and Veterans
    - *Patterns of Illness and Care Before Deployment to the Persian Gulf War*
    - Long-Term Follow-Up of Army Personnel Potentially Exposed to Chemical Warfare Agents
    - *Gulf War and Health: Infectious Diseases*
- Minority Health
    - Review and Assessment of the National Institutes of Health's Strategic Research Plan to Reduce and Ultimately Eliminate Health Disparities
    - Institutional and Policy-Level Strategies for Increasing the Racial and Ethnic Diversity of the U.S. Healthcare Workforce
    - *Communications for Behavior Change in the Twenty-First Century: Improving the Health of Diverse Populations*
- Public Policy
    - Redesigning Health Insurance Performance Measures, Payment, and Performance Improvement Programs
    - Identifying and Preventing Medication Errors
- Environment
    - *Evaluating Measures of Health Benefits for Environmental, Health, and Safety Regulation*

    - *Ethical Issues in Housing-Related Health Hazard Research Involving Children, Youth, and Families*
- Global Health
    - *Emerging Microbial Threats to Health in the Twenty-First Century*
    - *Advances in Technology and the Prevention of Their Application to Next Generation Biowarfare Agents*
- Health Sciences
    - *Assessing the System for Protecting Human Research Participants*
    - *Assessing Interactions among Social, Behavioral, and Genetic Factors in Health*
- Health Care and Quality
    - Work Environment for Nurses and Patient Safety
    - Immunization Safety Review
- Women's Health
    - Improving Mammography Quality Standards
    - Impact of Pregnancy Weight on Maternal and Child Health: A Workshop
- Treatment
    - Use of Complementary and Alternative Medicine (CAM) by the American Public
    - Spinal Cord Injury: Strategies in a Search for a Cure
- Workplace
    - Review of NIOSH (National Institute for Occupational Safety and Health) Hearing Loss Research Program
    - Asbestos: Selected Health Effects

### Cross-Cultural Education

Cross-cultural education and diversity training have gotten a great deal of attention. It is clear, however, that not enough has been done or the wrong approach has been used, for major disparities persist. Every nursing program needs to re-evaluate the content and experiences provided to the students. Every course can include cross-cultural issues.

There is a growing literature from which students can learn more about how diversity affects care and about different cultures. Films and television that include cultural issues can stimulate discussion. Every sector where disparities occur should be highlighted for students. Why does one patient receive care but not another? What is the impact of having no insurance? Do staff respond to minorities differently? Does the student respond differently? How does health literacy impact healthcare disparity? These questions will require a learning environment in which students feel comfortable being honest and responding without fear that their grades will be affected or that they will be criticized. They need an open environment, and faculty who will listen to them and guide them to a greater understanding. Clinical conferences are good occasions to address these questions. Use case-based learning that reflects cultural diversity—ethnicity, race, religion, family values—to help students reflect on how the growing diversity needs to be incorporated into care. A Muslim may want to pray seven times a day; a Muslim woman may not allow a male nurse or physician to touch her. The students need to be exposed to these values and discuss how they can be accommodated in care.

**Future Implications**

Some predictions for the future of health care and nursing education include:

- Social justice content required in nursing curricula
- Family history and genetic information incorporated into nursing health assessment
- More emphasis on health outcomes; measurement of the impact of nursing care on outcomes
- Emphasis on informatics throughout nursing curricula
- Shift to patient-centered care instead of institution-centered care
- Quality indicators used in nursing education to measure quality of care and quality improvement
- Access to care and the financing of care incorporated in all levels of nursing education in relation to nursing care reimbursement for services and impact of nursing shortage on access
- More funding for nursing education and partnerships with clinical and corporate entities to combat the nursing shortage
- Wider use of technology in health care, reflected in education
- Increased funding to improve access to nursing education and remove barriers to quality education
- Greater use of email, web-based patient education, and access to nurses and physicians via Internet
- Spirituality, mind and body, or integrative approaches to care incorporated in nursing education
- Increased lifespans, living with chronic illness; more emphasis on prevention, health promotion, disease management, financing
- Nursing's role redefined; work delegated to other healthcare professionals; more technology
- Flexible shifts, creative use of older nurses
- Greater use of simulation labs for interdisciplinary training
- Economic models incorporated into clinical agencies, nursing education
- Nurses more involved in wellness, stress management

## *Classroom Activities*

Many classroom and clinical learning activities are highlighted in Part 3, and others appear in the presentations described here. The following are other activities that can be incorporated in courses or clinical experiences.

### Story Sharing

Reflective journaling can help students to see their progress, to ask questions of faculty, and to reflect on their interactions with patients and their families. It is a good stress reducer as well. Faculty can share their stories with students to bring the clinical setting to life, to bridge the gap between the classroom and clinical agency.

> *A female, age 37, in relatively good health, with a history of a nonproductive cough for one week. Over-the-counter cough medications are not helping. She emails her primary healthcare provider for suggestions. He returns the email at the end of the day and states that he will order two prescriptions for her: one as a cough suppressant, the other to decrease inflammation. He will call in the prescription to the pharmacy. An hour later she receives a call from the pharmacy to confirm whether she is allergic to codeine. If so, can she take any amount of it without side effects? The answer is no. With this information they decide to call the physician because one of the medications contains codeine and he must change the order.*

Have the students discuss how this medication error could have occurred and how the new physician order entry system and integrated pharmacy dispensing system prevented the error. Most students can relate to this scenario, and therefore will engage in more lively dialogue about the role of the nurse, the health literacy of the patient, the use of informatics in patient care, and the impact of the IOM reports on health care.

### A Case Study

A 70-year-old woman with a history of irritable bowel syndrome (IBS) developed diarrhea for three weeks. She immediately called her physician and was seen. He prescribed a round of steroids for six days. The steroids made her feel better, but did little for the diarrhea. By week three she had lost about 15 pounds and was still cramping and having a little blood tinge to her stools. She went to see her physician, who ordered a CT scan and lab work. Two days later the lab work was still not ready, and she was getting weaker, unable to sleep, with diarrhea five to seven times per day. She was able to keep little food down because it caused diarrhea. She was drinking fluids with potassium and other electrolytes. The CT scan was still pending because the insurance company refused to pay for it. Preauthorization was needed, and the company did not view this as necessary medical treatment. As the nurse what should you consider?

- Age of the patient
- Medical history
- Bloody diarrhea
- Possible dehydration and electrolyte imbalance

- Possible ulcerative colitis
- Possible cancer
- Possible shifting of fluids due to steroids
- Possible false feeling of getting better due to steroids
- Impact of reimbursement process on treatment process and decisions (quality and safety)

### Root Cause Analysis

Use the case of the error in medication with codeine as the object of a root cause analysis. This means the problem is to be considered a systems failure and not an individual one. So what is happening? The physician pulls up the patient's electronic medical record. He notes that she has not been treated before for this problem. She is on no medications. Allergies do not appear on the record. He orders the medication with codeine and sends the order electronically to the pharmacy. The pharmacist pulls up the order on the screen and immediately gets a pop up window with an alert that says the patient is allergic to codeine. "If this order is to be processed you must document that you have read this alert and overridden the system." The pharmacist tries to reach the physician, who has gone home for the day. So the pharmacist calls the patient, who confirms that she is allergic to even the smallest amounts of codeine. So the pharmacist sends an email to the physician's office, and another physician changes the order. What is the cause of the problem? The system of medication allergy alerts worked in the pharmacy. Why then did it fail in the physician's office? The pharmacist and physician go back over the record and discover that in fact the allergies do appear on the physician office record, yet the order did not trigger an alert when it was placed. A computer glitch is found to be the problem, and the computer technician fixes it. All the physician's records are then checked to determine if this is an isolated incident or an officewide software problem. It is determined that it is isolated to this particular record. Possible safeguards are discussed with the office staff and physicians to avoid such an error in the future. One solution is to double check allergies before an order is sent to the pharmacy instead of relying on the computerized alert system.

### Steps in Critical Thinking

Critical thinking is a method of rationally considering the possible solutions to a problem. It questions what is seen or known within a context of what is real versus perceived. There are five steps in the critical thinking process:

1. Adopt the attitude of a critical thinker.
2. Recognize and avoid critical thinking hindrances.
3. Identify and characterize arguments.
4. Evaluate information sources.
5. Evaluate arguments. (Haskins, 2005)

This process is similar to the research or nursing process. Students must view themselves as detectives and question everything (attitude). Next, they must recognize the barriers that stand in the way of getting accurate information, for example, lack of medical history on the chart or inability of the patient to communicate clearly about current health problems. The third step is to recognize and identify the pros and cons of the situation. The fourth step is to determine if the source or sources are reliable. Finally, evaluate the conclusions drawn to determine whether every possibility has been considered or if there still is missing information that may affect the conclusion.

A man faints on an airplane when he abruptly stands up. After a few seconds he comes to and is able to talk to the flight crew. His color is pale, but lips and mucus membranes are pink. Why did he collapse?

1. Adopt the attitude. Look at the data. Assess the situation. The man is of average height and weight. No obvious problems. No clue yet as to the source of the problem.
2. Consider barriers to the problem. You ask the man for more information. What happened? How do you feel now? He states that he is okay and attempts to stand, obviously embarrassed. He faints again. Again he comes around in a few seconds. The barriers are his embarrassment and the presence of fellow passengers staring at him; the lack of medical equipment could be seen as another barrier. You ask him if he has any medical conditions, he says yes, high blood pressure. You ask if he is on medication, he says yes. When did he take it last? This morning (about eight hours ago). You are in a plane, so you ask how long he has been flying, he says about six hours.
3. Identify possible causes and consider the data so far: healthy-appearing man, good oxygenation by color, history of high blood pressure and nothing else, on medication, has been flying for several hours. What other factors do you consider? Flying dehydrates a person; antihypertensive medications alter blood circulation, which is also affected by flying; pressurization of the cabin affects the circulatory system; little food or fluids are given on planes; alcohol is available. You ask, has he had any alcohol? Yes, one and a half glasses of wine. You take a pulse, which is thready, but then stabilizes as you are talking.
4. You evaluate the source of your information. He seems reliable, and you trust your observations.
5. What is the problem? He might be dehydrated: the combination of little food and water, alcohol consumption, and flying, added to his medication, will deplete the body of fluids. You suggest that he be given water to drink. In three to five minutes he is able to stand without assistance and walk back to his seat.

## *Discussion Questions and Essay Questions*

### *1. Determinants of Health*

*How do the Healthy People 2010 determinants of health affect health care?* Select one healthcare problem (focus area) and apply: physical environment such as secondhand smoke, and cancer or asthma in children (pediatrics); how some groups in the population receive less care than others (racial and ethnic disparities); development of new mother support groups and education for high risk mothers (social connectedness and health; OB and pediatrics).

### *2. Chronic Illnesses*

The priority areas for action focus on chronic illness. Most healthcare resources (financial, staff, equipment) today are used for treatment of these problems. This care requires collaboration. Most of the care is provided by the patient or family. At this time the healthcare delivery system is not very effective in meeting the needs of these populations. It is not process-oriented and does not emphasize interdisciplinary teams and self-management, both of which are important in responding to chronic illnesses. Ask students the following:

- *What is your reaction to working with patients who have chronic illnesses? Would you do this work? Why or why not?*
- *What is the impact of chronic illness on the community?* (Students should consider issues such as lost work time, costs, transportation needs, impact on family, or long-term health, and their impact on quality of life and lifetime earning power.)
- *Do you know anyone with chronic illness? How do they feel about it? How has it affected their lives and those of their families? What difference would it make to you if the patient with a chronic illness were a child instead of an adult?*
- *If you were working with a patient population in the community that had a chronic illness, how might you use Healthy People 2010 to develop a plan of care for the population?*

### *3. Quality of Care*

*Describe the IOM report framework for healthcare quality. How can it be applied to nursing?*

### *4. Healthcare Safety*

- *Describe the IOM report framework for healthcare safety. How it might be applied to nursing?*
- *What is your opinion of a "No Blame" culture? How might this be applied in your school environment? In a hospital environment?*
- *Why is lifelong learning necessary to improve health care? Provide specific examples.*

***5. Informatics***

*What are the implications of the following statement: medical technology has moved nursing care away from caring in practice into an age where there is greater quality and safety and patients are more satisfied?*

***6. Workplace Safety***

*Ask students to select an ANA publication on workplace safety (at http://www.nursingworld.org), review the document, and discuss implications.*

## Self-Assessment Tools

Self-assessment tools can be used to determine how well a particular problem has been solved, such as an emergency response to a public health issue. Columbia University offers an online course that lets students review content about emergency response and participate in a self-assessment (http://cpmcnet.columbia.edu/dept/nursing/institute-centers/chphsr/ERMain.html). Similar assessment tools developed by ANA are used by clinical agencies. These include: *Implementing Nursing's Report Card: A Study of RN Staffing, Length of Stay, and Patient Outcomes; NIDSEC: Standards and Scoring Guidelines; Nursing Care Report Card for Acute Care; Nursing Quality Indicators Beyond Acute Care: Literature Review; Nursing Quality Indicators Beyond Acute Care: Measurement Instruments; Nursing Quality Indicators Set; Nursing Quality Indicators: Definitions and Implications; Nursing Quality Indicators: Guide for Implementation;* and *Nursing Quality Measurement: A Review of Nursing Studies.*

Several nursing education self-assessment tools can help initiate a continuous quality improvement plan and ongoing evaluation. These take in curricular or faculty evaluations as well as business processes, mainly in relationship to student services.

The University of Oklahoma Health Sciences Center College of Nursing uses a commercial online course evaluation system that can be customized to include information about the course content. If the course uses technology or technical support, it can record how well they performed. Beyond these typical course evaluation functions, computerized data collection on all courses, including face-to-face courses, allows the student cohort to be tracked over their academic program. Faculty evaluations are also computerized and put into a database to allow comparisons of faculty effectiveness across teaching modalities or sections of students.

Self-assessment technology can be used to link course and faculty evaluation data to admissions data from a student database. If a student is not doing well, a root cause analysis may uncover factors that indicate a need for tutoring or intensive English classes. This database allows student admission, academic progress, and graduation to be tracked and services improved.

End-of-program evaluations reveal how well students think their program went and what changes, if any, they would suggest. There are many commercial products available.

Alumni surveys can obtain information about strengths and weaknesses of the educational program a year after graduation, when the student has had a chance to apply what was learned.

Ongoing student evaluations support testing at key points in the curriculum and then remediation in weak areas. If many of the best students are struggling in a certain area, then the content is probably not being covered effectively.

Overall services can also be benchmarked against peer institutions that use the same commercial service. Elements include student advising, student tutoring, staff availability, technical support for admission, registration, progression, graduation processes, ability of staff or faculty to answer student questions, and usability of information (paper or online; admission, progression policies, or graduation information). These evaluations furnish the educational institution with a report card on its services. It helps the institution improve or maintain excellent services, while root cause analysis helps restore quality where the system has failed.

## *Questions for Reflection*

It is not too soon to think about the long-term repercussions of the IOM reports for nursing education. Some questions to consider:

- What will the role of the nurse be in 2020?
- What will healthcare delivery look like in 2020?
- Given the aging population and dwindling resources, what types of services should we be considering today to improve health outcomes in 2020?
- Will the United States adopt a national health insurance plan by 2020?
- What are the long-range nursing or health care policy implications of the IOM reports?
- How will technology influence health care in 2020?

## *Teaching IOM: Test Questions*

These include multiple-choice and essay questions. The answers start on page 75.

### Exam Questions

The following questions cover material in the five PowerPoint presentations found on the CD-ROM.

1. **In patient-centered care the key focus is best described as:**
   a. Patients describing how they feel about past treatment and expectations
   b. The nurse completing a nursing assessment in a timely manner
   c. The hospital asking patients if they have an advanced directive
   d. Patients being told in the ER that they must contact their insurer

2. **Which of the following is the best description of evidence-based practice?**
    a. Use of research results when approved by a professional body
    b. Integrating best research results, clinical expertise, and patient values
    c. Applying research results by healthcare practitioner
    d. Documenting rationales for treatment decisions by using research results
3. **Which of the following is considered to be a component of the healthcare quality dimension?**
    a. Staying healthy
    b. Living with illness or disability
    c. Timeliness
    d. Getting better
4. **Three criteria are used to identify the priority areas of health care. Which of the following is not one of the criteria?**
    a. Impact
    b. Improvability
    c. Consumer view of importance
    d. Inclusiveness
5. **Which of the following would not be considered an important strategy for reducing disparity in health care?**
    a. Offer universal healthcare coverage.
    b. Focus more on insurance coverage rather than access and efficiency.
    c. Increase representation of minorities in the health professions.
    d. Increase the amount of content and learning experiences about disparity for staff.
6. **Who are the some of the stakeholders in the quality initiative?**
    a. Patient
    b. Employers
    c. Nurse
    d. All of the above
7. **Which of these factors has had a particular impact on the quality of health care?**
    a. Cost of care
    b. Increase in chronic illnesses
    c. Number of healthcare providers
    d. Efficiency within the system
8. **You are a nurse working in a rural community. The community appears to have a high rate of cardiac disease. You are preparing a plan to address this need. Which of the following is a critical resource as you develop your plan?**
    a. *The Sullivan Commission Report*
    b. *Healthy People 2010*
    c. World Health Organization
    d. *The National Healthcare Quality Report*

9. **You are a hospital nurse on the quality team. The team is developing a list of focus areas for the annual review of quality. The team is using the national priority areas of care as its guide. Which of the following would not belong on the list?**
   a. Care coordination
   b. Diabetes
   c. GI problems
   d. Nosocomial infections
10. **The National Healthcare Disparities Report includes which information that is part of other critical healthcare delivery reports?**
    a. Staying healthy, getting better, living with illness and disability, coping with end of life
    b. Cost of care per disease category and treatment offered
    c. Error rate and identification of type of error and who makes the error
    d. Health professions education needs
11. **Which report focuses on disparity in the nation's health professional workforce?**
    a. *To Err Is Human*
    b. *Health Professions Education*
    c. *The Sullivan Commission Report*
    d. *Crossing the Quality Chasm*
12. **A nurse is preparing medications and puts the wrong medication on the tray for a patient. Before she enters the room she looks at the medication and realizes it is the wrong color and returns to check the medication bottle. She reports this to nurse manager as a near miss. What is the most appropriate explanation of the importance of a near miss?**
    a. Near misses are common in healthcare delivery.
    b. Identifying near misses can reduce healthcare costs.
    c. Willingness to identify near misses indicates safety is valued, part of the culture.
    d. Increased education can decrease near misses.
13. **Mrs. Jones has been noncompliant with her treatment at home for diabetes. Under what circumstance might noncompliance be considered an error?**
    a. Mrs. Jones calls the doctor when she has a respiratory infection.
    b. Mrs. Jones decides she needs to decrease her insulin to save money.
    c. Mrs. Jones checks her blood sugar levels but is confused about the results.
    d. Mrs. Jones exercises every other day.
14. **Which of the following is causing the most concern today about errors in healthcare delivery?**
    a. Review of medical records
    b. Mandatory reporting
    c. Automated surveillance
    d. Education of healthcare professionals about errors

15. **A patient is admitted for surgery and while in the hospital develops a urinary infection while an urinary catheter is inserted, which increases his hospital stay by 3 days. What type of error is this?**
    a. Active
    b. Latent
    c. Error of planning
    d. Iatrogenic
16. **You are a nurse working in a community clinic and need information that can guide treatment for patients with asthma. Where would you quickly find clinical guidelines about asthma?**
    a. Foundation for Accountability web site
    b. National Center for Nursing Quality web site
    c. Agency for Healthcare Research and Quality web site
    d. Medicare web site
17. **One of the most recent efforts to improve care and practice, which has had an impact on how care is viewed and evaluated, is:**
    a. The Magnet Hospital Recognition Program
    b. JCAHO accreditation process
    c. NLN accreditation of schools of nursing
    d. The Leapfrog Group
18. **The National Healthcare Quality Report includes all of the following except:**
    a. Data about patient perspectives
    b. A collection of individual hospital report cards
    c. Healthcare delivery system performance
    d. Accessible data
19. **The services provided in a city healthcare clinic system are assessed. Some groups of the population have less timely access to certain diagnostic tests, although their condition warrants these tests. This might best be described as:**
    a. Stereotypes
    b. Patient preferences
    c. Discrimination
    d. Efficient delivery
20. **The nursing staff on a unit are discussing a recent error which resulted in the patient going to ICU and being intubated for 2 weeks. They need to analyze what occurred. What is the best description of the type of error?**
    a. Near miss
    b. Latent error
    c. Sentinel event
    d. Diagnostic
21. **The IOM reports have identified new rules for healthcare delivery. Which of the following is a current rule and not a new rule?**
    a. Transparency is necessary.
    b. Decision-making is evidence based.

c. The patient is the source of control.
d. Cost reduction is sought.

22. **The National Healthcare Quality Report contains data organized by states.**
    a. True
    b. False
23. **JCAHO accreditation requires hospitals to meet specific standards in a specific manner.**
    a. True
    b. False
24. **The best approach to assessing quality of care is to include as many diseases and their treatment as possible to reach the best view of the status of healthcare delivery.**
    a. True
    b. False
25. **A new rule in the twenty-first century healthcare system is that professional autonomy drives variability in care.**
    a. True
    b. False
26. **The goal of public health is to assist those without insurance.**
    a. True
    b. False
27. **An error in a surgical procedure is which type of error?**
    a. Preventive
    b. Diagnostic
    c. General
    d. Treatment
28. **The public health nurse should spend time on empowering those who live in the community.**
    a. True
    b. False
29. **Access to care focuses on entry into the system and within the system.**
    a. True
    b. False
30. **Safe care is quality care.**
    a. True
    b. False

### Short Essay Questions

1. Discuss three reasons why errors are often not documented.
2. Describe the culture of blame and how it affects healthcare delivery.
3. Explain the root cause analysis process.
4. Identify two current JCAHO safety goals and explain how they affect your practice.

5. Explain what is meant by disparity in health care.
6. Discuss the impact of uninsurance and underinsurance on healthcare delivery.
7. Describe the public health core functions, providing examples, and what impact they have on the nation's public health.
8. Select two of the six improvement aims, discuss what they mean, and describe an example from your experience.
9. How does globalization affect public health?
10. Select two of the core competencies for healthcare professionals and defend why these should be core competencies for all healthcare professionals. Support your answer with examples.
11. Compare the two dimensions of the National Healthcare Quality Report Matrix.
12. Discuss why you might use the Forces of Magnetism in a search for a new job.

## *Exam Questions with Correct Answers*

1. **In patient-centered care the key focus is best described as:**
   a. Patients describing how they feel about past treatment and expectations
   b. The nurse completing a nursing assessment in a timely manner
   c. The hospital asking patients if they have an advanced directive
   d. Patients being told in the ER that they must contact their insurer

   *a. Patient-centered care begins with and focuses on how the patient views their illness and healthcare received or not received. This information then is used to guide care provided.*

2. **Which of the following is the best description of evidence-based practice?**
   a. Use of research results when approved by a professional body
   b. Integrating best research results, clinical expertise, and patient values
   c. Applying research results by healthcare practitioner
   d. Documenting rationales for treatment decisions by using research results

   *b. This statement includes the critical elements: best research results indicating that there has been an evaluation of results, the expertise of the healthcare provider, and the patient.*

3. **Which of the following is considered to be a component of the healthcare quality dimension?**
   a. Staying healthy
   b. Living with illness or disability
   c. Timeliness
   d. Getting better

   *c. The other three responses are components of consumer perspectives on healthcare needs.*

4. **Three criteria are used to identify the priority areas of health care. Which of the following is not one of the criteria?**
   a. Impact
   b. Improvability
   c. Consumer view of importance
   d. Inclusiveness

   *c. Consumers are important, but their view of importance is not one of the criteria.*

5. **Which of the following would not be considered an important strategy for reducing disparity in health care?**
   a. Offer universal healthcare coverage.
   b. Focus more on insurance coverage rather than access and efficiency.
   c. Increase representation of minorities in the health professions.
   d. Increase the amount of content and learning experiences about disparity for staff.

   *b. Insurance coverage is very important, but we must consider how patients get care independent of how they will pay for it. Many people have Medicaid and Medicare but still have problems finding physicians to see them, getting clinic appointments, and so on.*

6. **Who are the some of the stakeholders in the quality initiative?**
   a. Patient
   b. Employers
   c. Nurse
   d. All of the above

   *d. All of these are stakeholders; others are insurers, family members, government, pharmaceutical companies, other healthcare providers, and medical supply and equipment resources.*

7. **Which of these factors has had a particular impact on the quality of health care?**
   a. Cost of care
   b. Increase in chronic illnesses
   c. Number of healthcare providers
   d. Efficiency within the system

   *b. The increase of chronic illness has had an impact on health care. Patients with chronic illnesses particularly require a healthcare system that is consistent, accessible, and easy to use.*

8. **You are a nurse working in a rural community. The community appears to have a high rate of cardiac disease. You are preparing a plan to address**

**this need. Which of the following is a critical resource as you develop your plan?**

a. *The Sullivan Commission Report*
b. *Healthy People 2010*
c. World Health Organization
d. *The National Healthcare Quality Report*

*b. Healthy People 2010 is accessible on the Internet and identifies key goals and objectives for specific health problems such as cardiac disease and offers current data related to the goals and objectives that communities can use to improve the health of the community members.*

9. **You are a hospital nurse on the quality team. The team is developing a list of focus areas for the annual review of quality. The team is using the national priority areas of care as its guide. Which of the following would not belong on the list?**
   a. Care coordination
   b. Diabetes
   c. GI problems
   d. Nosocomial infections

   *c. GI problems is not on the current list of priority problems.*

10. **The National Healthcare Disparities Report includes which information that is part of other critical healthcare delivery reports?**
    a. Staying healthy, getting better, living with illness and disability, coping with end-of-life
    b. Cost of care per disease category and treatment offered
    c. Error rate and identification of type of error and who makes the error
    d. Health professions education needs

    *a. These elements are found in the National Quality Report, which emphasizes the consumer perspectives.*

11. **Which report focuses on disparity in the nation's health professional workforce?**
    a. *To Err Is Human*
    b. *Health Professions Education*
    c. *The Sullivan Commission Report*
    d. *Crossing the Quality Chasm*

    *c. The Sullivan Commission explored the need to consider the number of minorities in healthcare disparity.*

12. **A nurse is preparing medications and puts the wrong medication on the tray for a patient. Before she enters the room she looks at the medication**

**and realizes it is the wrong color and returns to check the medication bottle. She reports this to nurse manager as a near miss. What is the most appropriate explanation of the importance of a near miss?**

a. Near misses are common in healthcare delivery.
b. Identifying near misses can reduce healthcare costs.
c. Willingness to identify near misses indicates safety is valued, part of the culture.
d. Increased education can decrease near misses.

*c. Staff who report near misses feel comfortable that they will not be automatically blamed and that the organization has a culture in which safety is valued.*

13. **Mrs. Jones has been noncompliant with her treatment at home for diabetes. Under what circumstance might noncompliance be considered an error?**

a. Mrs. Jones calls the doctor when she has a respiratory infection.
b. Mrs. Jones decides she needs to decrease her insulin to save money.
c. Mrs. Jones checks her blood sugar levels but is confused about the results.
d. Mrs. Jones exercises every other day.

*b. Mrs. Jones is not making a decision about her insulin based on sound self-management of her care that requires she follow the prescription for insulin. Decreasing insulin for cost reasons is noncompliance. She needs help in finding resources for her treatment so that she can be compliant.*

14. **Which of the following is causing the most concern today about errors in healthcare delivery?**

a. Review of medical records
b. Mandatory reporting
c. Automated surveillance
d. Education of healthcare professionals about errors

*b. Healthcare professionals are concerned most about mandatory reporting of errors. They are concerned about possible implications, for example, malpractice and impacts on their jobs.*

15. **A patient is admitted for surgery and while in the hospital develops a urinary infection while an urinary catheter is inserted, which increases his hospital stay by 3 days. What type of error is this?**

a. Active
b. Latent
c. Error of planning
d. Iatrogenic

*d. Iatrogenic injury occurs when harm to the patient is caused by or originates from care management.*

16. **You are a nurse working in a community clinic and need information that can guide treatment for patients with asthma. Where would you quickly find clinical guidelines about asthma?**
    a. Foundation for Accountability web site
    b. National Center for Nursing Quality web site
    c. Agency for Healthcare Research and Quality web site
    d. Medicare web site

    *c. AHRQ is the site of the National Clearinghouse for clinical guidelines.*

17. **One of the most recent efforts to improve care and practice, which has had an impact on how care is viewed and evaluated, is:**
    a. The Magnet Hospital Recognition Program
    b. JCAHO accreditation process
    c. NLN accreditation of schools of nursing
    d. The Leapfrog Group

    *a. The Magnet program has helped to clarify the critical elements of higher quality and safer care through its identification of the forces of magnetism. JCAHO and NLN accreditations are not new. The Leapfrog Group is new but it is made up mostly of employers concerned about health care; it may make an impact but is not as important as the Magnet program is now.*

18. **The National Healthcare Quality Report includes all of the following except:**
    a. Data about patient perspectives
    b. A collection of individual hospital report cards
    c. Healthcare delivery system performance
    d. Accessible data

    *b. The report should not duplicate efforts by individual hospitals to describe the quality of their care in report cards.*

19. **The services provided in a city healthcare clinic system are assessed. Some groups of the population have less timely access to certain diagnostic tests although their condition warrants these tests. This might best be described as:**
    a. Stereotypes
    b. Patient preferences
    c. Discrimination
    d. Efficient delivery

    *c. Discrimination means differences in care that result from biases, prejudices, stereotyping, or uncertainty in clinical communication and decision-making.*

20. **The nursing staff on a unit are discussing a recent error which resulted in the patient going to ICU and being intubated for 2 weeks. They need**

**to analyze what occurred. What is the best description of the type of error?**

a. Near miss
b. Latent error
c. Sentinel event
d. Diagnostic

*c. This is a sentinel event, which is an unexpected occurrence involving death or serious physical or psychological injury or risk of this. It is not a near miss, as the error did occur; it is not latent, as it did cause harm; it could be related to a diagnostic error, but based on information provided this is unknown at this time. A sentinel event must always be analyzed so that care can improve.*

**21. The IOM reports have identified new rules for healthcare delivery. Which of the following is a current rule and not a new rule?**

a. Transparency is necessary.
b. Decision-making is evidence based.
c. The patient is the source of control.
d. Cost reduction is sought.

*d. Cost reduction is important, but now there is greater emphasis on waste reduction as a way to decrease costs.*

**22. The National Healthcare Quality Report contains data organized by states.**

a. True
b. False

*a. Data related to specific states can be found in the annual report about the nation's health care.*

**23. JCAHO accreditation requires hospitals to meet specific standards in a specific manner.**

a. True
b. False

*b. JCAHO has moved away from rigid standards, allowing more flexibility in how a standard is met as long as certain principles are followed.*

**24. The best approach to assessing quality of care is to include as many diseases and their treatment as possible to reach the best view of the status of healthcare delivery.**

a. True
b. False

*b. It is not practical to effectively analyze as many diseases and their treatment as possible; it takes too many resources and may miss something. The priority areas of care help to focus the analysis and are chosen for their importance.*

25. **A new rule in the twenty-first century healthcare system is that professional autonomy drives variability in care.**
   a. True
   b. False

   *b. This the current rule, but the new rule is that care is customized according to patient values and needs, which supports patient-centered care.*

26. **The goal of public health is to assist those without insurance.**
   a. True
   b. False

   *b. Public health has an impact on all members of the community, and the goal is to improve the public's health, for example, immunizations, nutrition, and environmental health (water, air, etc.), safety.*

27. **An error in a surgical procedure is which type of error?**
   a. Preventive
   b. Diagnostic
   c. General
   d. Treatment

   *d. A treatment error is an error in performance of a procedure or an avoidable delay in treatment.*

28. **The public health nurse should spend time on empowering those who live in the community.**
   a. True
   b. False

   *a. Empowerment is one of the essential public health services; community members need to know how to speak up for themselves and participate actively in expressing their needs and evaluating the public health services they receive.*

29. **Access to care focuses on entry into the system and within the system.**
   a. True
   b. False

   *a. Both components are important to reach maximum access for patients.*

30. **Safe care is quality care.**
   a. True
   b. False

   *b. Safe care means there is a greater chance that the care is of higher quality, but care can be safe and not of higher quality.*

# Part 5

# References, Readings, Internet Sites, and Other Resources

This part of the book consolidates all the references from the main part of the text along with other resources that instructors and students can use for further study. Its contents are grouped into these four sections:

- Online Access to IOM Reports
- References for Parts 1 through 4 and the Glossary
- Additional Readings
- Additional References: Evidence-Based Practice and Research

The URLs noted in these pages were retrieved and verified as of July 2006.

## Online Access to IOM Reports

You can also access these and all other IOM reports issued since 1998, or download a list of all reports since 1970, at the IOM home page (http://www.iom.edu) by choosing "Reports."


*To Err Is Human: Building A Safer Health System.* (1999). http://www.iom.edu/report.asp?id=5575.

*Crossing the Quality Chasm.* (2001). http://www.iom.edu/report.asp?id=5432.

*Envisioning the National Health Care Quality.* (2001). http://www.iom.edu/report.asp?id=5441.

*Guidance for the National Healthcare Disparities Report.* (2002). http://www.iom.edu/report.asp?id=4353.

*Unequal Treatment: Confronting Racial and Ethnic Disparities in Health Care.* (2002). http://www.iom.edu/report.asp?id=4475.

*Health Professions Education: A Bridge to Quality.* (2003). http://www.iom.edu/report.asp?id=5914.

*The Future of the Public's Health in the 21st Century.* (2003). http://www.iom.edu/CMS/3793/4720/4304.aspx.
*Keeping Patients Safe: Transforming the Work Environment for Nurses.* (2003). http://www.iom.edu/report.asp?id=16173.
*Leadership By Example: Coordinating Government Roles in Improving Health Care Quality.* (2003). http://www.iom.edu/report.asp?id=4309.
*Patient Safety: Achieving a New Standard for Care.* (2003). http://www.iom.edu/report.asp?id=16663.
*Priority Areas for National Action: Transforming Health Care Quality.* (2003). http://www.iom.edu/report.asp?id=4290.
*Who Will Keep the Public Healthy?.* (2003). http://www.nap.edu/books/030908542X/htm.
*Health Literacy: A Prescription to End Confusion.* (2004). http://www.iom.edu/report.asp?id=19723.

## *References: Part 1*

American Association of Colleges of Nursing (AACN). (1998). *The essentials of baccalaureate education for professional nursing practice.* Washington, DC: AACN.
Berwick, D. (2003, April). *Pursuing perfection: Raising the bar for healthcare performance.* Learning Network Meeting, Boston, MA. Cambridge, MA: Institute for Healthcare Improvement.
Donabedian, A. (1980). *Explorations in quality assessment and monitoring* (Vol. 1). Ann Arbor, MI: Health Administration Press.
Donabedian, A. (1996). Evaluating the quality of medical care. *Milbank Quarterly, 44,* 166–203.
Institute of Medicine (IOM). (1990). *Medicare: A strategy for quality assurance.* Washington, DC: National Academies Press.
Institute of Medicine (IOM). (1999). *To err is human: Building a safer health system.* Washington, DC: Institute of Medicine and National Academies Press.
Institute of Medicine (IOM). (2001a). *Crossing the quality chasm.* Washington, DC: National Academies Press.
Institute of Medicine (IOM). (2001b). *Envisioning the national health care quality.* Washington, DC: National Academies Press.
Institute of Medicine (IOM). (2002a). *Unequal treatment: Confronting racial and ethnic disparities in health.* Washington, DC: National Academies Press.
Institute of Medicine (IOM). (2002b). *Guidance for the national healthcare disparities report.* Washington, DC: National Academies Press.
Institute of Medicine (IOM). (2003a). *Priority areas for national action: Transforming health care quality.* Washington, DC: National Academies Press.
Institute of Medicine (IOM). (2003b). *Leadership by example: Coordinating government roles in improving health care.* Washington, DC: National Academies Press.

Institute of Medicine (IOM). (2003c). *The future of the public's health in the 21st century*. Washington, DC: National Academies Press.
Institute of Medicine (IOM). (2003d). *Who will keep the public healthy*? Washington, DC: National Academies Press.
Institute of Medicine (IOM). (2003e). *Health professions education: A bridge to quality.* Washington, DC: National Academies Press.
Institute of Medicine (IOM). (2004a). *Keeping patients safe: Transforming the work environment for nurses*. Washington, DC: National Academies Press.
Institute of Medicine (IOM). (2004b). *Patient safety: Achieving a new standard of care.* Washington, DC: National Academies Press.
Long, K. (2003). The Institute of Medicine report *Health professions education: A bridge to quality. Policy, politics, & nursing practice,* *4*(4): 259–262.
McClosky, J., & Bulechek, G. (Eds.). (2000). *Nursing interventions classification.* St. Louis, MO: Mosby, Inc.
Scalise, D. (2005). Patient care: The safety network. *Hospitals & Health Networks, 79*(12), 16–17.
Sullivan, L. W. (2004). *Missing persons: Minorities in the health professions: A report of the Sullivan Commission on diversity in the healthcare workforces.* http://64.233.167.104/search?q=cache:MHACBuil7LUJ:www.aacn.nche.edu/SullivanReport.pdf+sullivan+commission+report+on+health+disparities&hl=en. Accessed 01/02/05.
The President's Advisory Commission on Consumer Protection and Quality in the Healthcare Industry. (1999). *Quality first: Better healthcare for all Americans.* Washington, DC: U.S. Government Printing Office.
Wakefield, M. (1997). Pioneering new ways to ensure quality healthcare. *Nursing Economics, 15*(4), 225–227.

## References: Parts 2 and 3

Agency for Healthcare Research and Quality (AHRQ). (2003). *AHRQ's patient safety initiative: Building foundations, reducing risk.* Interim Report to the Senate Committee on Appropriations. AHRQ Publication No. 04-RG005, December, 2003. Rockville, MD: Agency for Healthcare Research and Quality. http://www.ahrq.gov/qual/pscongrpt.
American Association of Colleges of Nursing (AACN). (1999). A vision of baccalaureate and graduate nursing education: The next decade. *Journal of Professional Nursing, 15*(1), 59–65.
American Association of Colleges of Nursing (AACN). (2003). *Clinical nurse leader.* White paper. Washington, DC: AACN.
American Association of Colleges of Nursing (AACN). (2005a). *The clinical nurse leader*[SM]*: Developing a new nursing role.* http://www.aacn.nche.edu/CNL/.
American Association of Colleges of Nursing (AACN). (2005b). *AACN Position statement on the practice doctorate in nursing,* October 2004. http://www.aacn.nche.edu/Education/index.htm. Accessed February 13, 2005.

Banister, G., Butt, L., & Hackel, R. (1996). How nurses perceive medication errors. *Nursing Management, 27*(1), 31–34.

Dunton, N., Gajewski, B., Taunton, R., & Moore, J. (2004). Nursing staffing and patient falls in acute care hospital units. *Nursing Outlook, 52*(1), 53–59.

Ignatavicius, D. (2000). Do you help staff rise to the fall prevention challenge? *Nursing Management,* (1), 27–30.

Institute of Medicine (IOM). (2001). *Crossing the quality chasm*. Washington, DC: National Academies Press.

Institute of Medicine (IOM). (2003a). *Health literacy: A prescription to end confusion.* Washington, DC: National Academies Press.

Institute of Medicine (IOM). (2003b). *Health professions education: A bridge to quality.* Washington, DC: National Academies Press.

Institute of Medicine (IOM). (2003c). *Priority areas for national action: Transforming health care quality*. Washington, DC: National Academies Press.

Institute of Medicine (IOM). (2004). *Keeping patients safe: Transforming the work environment for nurses.* Washington, DC: National Academies Press.

Jones, B. (2002). Nurses and the code of silence. In M. D. Rosenthal & K. M. Sutcliffe (Eds.), *Medical error: What do we know? What do we do?* San Francisco, CA: Jossey-Bass.

Jones, M. (2001). Medical errors. *Journal of Legal Nurse Consultants, 12*(3), 16–19.

Lamb, G., Jennings, B., Mitchell, P., & Lang, N. (2004). Quality agenda: Priorities for action recommendations of the American Academy of Nursing conference on healthcare quality. *Nursing Outlook, 52* (1), 60–65.

Locsin, R. (2005). *Technology competency as caring in nursing*. Indianapolis, IN: Sigma Theta Tau International.

Mark, B., Hughes, L., & Jones, C. (2004). The role of theory in improving patient safety and quality healthcare. *Nursing Outlook, 52*(1), 11–16.

McBride, A. B. (2005). Actually achieving our preferred future. *Reflections on Nursing Leadership, Fourth Quarter*, 22–23, 28.

McClure, M., & Hinshaw, A. (2002). *Magnet hospital revisited, forces of magnetism: Organizational elements of excellence in nursing care,* Washington, DC: American Nurses Publishing.

Michaelsen, L., Knight, A., & Fink, L. (2004). *Team-based learning: A transformative use of small groups in college teaching*. Sterling, VA: Stylus Publishing.

Shortell, S., Gillies, R., & Anderson, D. (2000). *Remaking healthcare in America* (2nd ed.). San Francisco, CA: Jossey-Bass.

Steefel, L. (2002). Nix medication errors the new-fashioned way. *Nursing Spectrum* (June), 26MW.

Stevens, K. R. (2005). *Essential competencies for evidence-based practice in nursing* (1st ed.). San Antonio, TX: The University of Texas Health Science Center at San Antonio.

Wrong Site Surgery Errors. *(2004). The American Nurse, 36*(1), 6.

## *References: Part 4*

See also the URLs for the specific reports under Online Access to IOM Reports on page 83.

Donabedian, A. (1996). Evaluating the quality of medical care. *Milbank Quarterly, 44,* 166–203.

Dovidio, J. et al. (1996). Stereotyping, prejudice, and discrimination: Another look. In N. Macrae, C. Stangor, & M. Hewstone (Eds.). *Stereotypes and stereotyping* (pp. 276–319). NY: Guilford.

Haskins, G. R. (2005). A practical guide to critical thinking. http://skepdic.com/essays/haskins.pdf.

Hundert, E., Hafferty, F., & Christakis, D. (1996). Characteristics of the informal curriculum and trainees' ethical choices. *Academic Medicine, 71*(6), 624–642.

U.S. Department of Health and Human Services (DHHS). (2000). *Healthy People 2010.* Washington, DC: U.S. Government Printing Office.

## *Additional Readings*

The readings in this section are a representative selection of the literature that addresses one or more of the issues discussed in this book.

Agency for Healthcare Research Quality (AHRQ). (2000). *Translating research into practice: From the pipeline of health services research-CAHPS.* The story of the consumer assessment of health plans. Online at http://www.ahrq.gov/research/cahptrip.htm.

Agency for Healthcare Research and Quality (AHRQ). (2001). *Making health care safer: A critical analysis of patient safety practices.* Evidence Report/Technology Assessment: Number 43. AHRQ Publication No. 01-E058. Rockville, MD: Agency for Healthcare Research and Quality. http://www.ahrq.gov/clinic/ptsafety/.

Agency for Healthcare Research and Quality (AHRQ). (2003). *AHRQ's patient safety initiative: Building foundations, reducing risk.* Interim Report to the Senate Committee on Appropriations. AHRQ Publication No. 04-RG005. Rockville, MD: Agency for Healthcare Research and Quality. http://www.ahrq.gov/qual/pscongrpt.

Agency for Healthcare Research and Quality (AHRQ). (2004). *Strategies for improving minority healthcare quality.* Evidence Report/Technology Assessment: Number 90. http:///www.ahrq.gov/clinic/epcsums/minqusum.htm.

AHRQ, IOM weigh in on developing a health-literate America. (2004). *Quality Letter for Healthcare Leaders, 16*(5), 6–8.

Aiken, L. H., Clarke, S. P., Cheung, R. B., Sloane, D. M., and Silber, J. (2003). Education levels of hospital nurses and patient mortality. *Journal of American Medical Association, 290*(12), 1–8.

Aiken, L. H., Clarke, S. P., Sloane, D. M., Sochalski, J., & Silber, J. H. (2002). Hospital nurse staffing and patient mortality, nurse burnout, and job dissatisfaction. *Journal of American Medical Association, 288*(16), 1987–1993.

Allan, J., Barwick, T. A., Cashman, S., Cawley, J. F., Day, C., Douglass, et al. (2004). Clinical prevention and population health: Curriculum framework for health professions. *American Journal of Preventive Medicine, 27*(5), 471–476.

American Association of Colleges of Nursing (AACN). (2002a). *Hallmarks of the professional nursing practice environment.* Washington, DC: AACN.

American Association of Colleges of Nursing (AACN). (2002b). *Nursing education's agenda for the 21st century.* Washington, DC: AACN.

American Association of Colleges of Nursing (AACN). (2002c). *Report of the task force on education and regulation.* Washington, DC: AACN.

American Association of Colleges of Nursing (AACN). (2002d). *Using strategic partnerships to expand nursing education programs.* Washington, DC: AACN.

American Association of Colleges of Nursing (AACN). (2003). *Building capacity through university hospital and university School of Nursing partnerships.* Washington, DC: AACN.

American College of Physicians (ACP). (2004). Racial and ethnic disparities in healthcare. A position paper of the American College of Physicians. *Annals of Internal Medicine, 141*(3), 226–232.

American Hospital Association (AHA), Commission on Workforce for Hospitals and Health Systems. (2002). *In our hands: How hospital leaders can build a thriving workforce.* Chicago: AHA.

American Medical Association (AMA). (2001). *Health literacy introductory kit.* http://www.ama-assn.org/ama/pub/category/8115.html.

American Nurses Association (ANA). (1995). *Nursing care report card for acute care.* Washington, DC: American Nurses Publishing.

American Nurses Association (ANA). (1996). *Nursing quality indicators.* Washington, DC: American Nurses Publishing.

American Nurses Association (ANA). (1997). *Implementing nursing's report card: A study of RN staffing, length of stay, and patient outcomes.* Washington, DC: American Nurses Publishing.

American Nurses Association (ANA). (1999a). *ANA's needlestick prevention guide.* http://www.nursingworld.org.

American Nurses Association (ANA). (1999b). *Nursing-sensitive quality indicators for acute care settings and ANA's safety and quality initiative.* http://www.nursingworld.org.

American Nurses Association (ANA). (2000). *Nursing staffing and patient outcomes in the inpatient hospital setting.* Washington, DC: American Nurses Publishing.

American Nurses Association (ANA). (2002a). *Preventing back injuries: Safe patient handling and movement.* http://www.nursingworld.org.

American Nurses Association (ANA). (2002b). *Preventing transmission of tuberculosis.* http://www.nursingworld.org.

American Nurses Association (ANA). (2002c). *Principles for documentation*. Washington, DC: ANA.

American Nurses Association (ANA). (2002d).*Your health and safety rights*. http://www.nursingworld.org.

American Nurses Association (ANA). (2003a). ANA House of Delegates status report: National database for nursing quality indicators. Washington, DC: ANA.

American Nurses Association (ANA). (2003b). *Principles for staffing*. Washington, DC: ANA.

Aydin, C. E., Bolton, L. B., Donaldson, N., Brown, D. S., Buffum, M., Elashoff, J. D., & Sandhu, M. (2004). Creating and analyzing a statewide nursing quality measurement database. *Journal of Nursing Scholarship, 36*(4), 371–378.

Baier, R. R., Kissam, S., & Gifford, D. R. (2005). Data's role in quality improvement. *Provider, 31*(1), 43–45.

Balas, M., Scott, L., & Rogers, A. (2004). The prevalence and nature of errors and near errors reported by hospital staff nurses. *Applied Nursing Research, 17*(4), 224–230.

Banister, G., Butt, L., & Hackel, R. (1996). How nurses perceive medication errors. *Nursing Management, 27*(1), 31–34.

Barger, S. E. (2004). Academic nursing centers: The road from the past, the bridge to the future. *Journal of Nursing Education, 43*(2), 60–65.

Bates, D., Teich, J. M., Lee, J., Seger, D., Kuperman, G. J., Ma'Luf, N.,et al. (1999). The impact of computerized physician order entry on medication error prevention. *Journal of American Medical Information Association, 6*(4), 313–321.

Bates-Jensen, B. (2001). Quality indicators for prevention and management of pressure ulcers in vulnerable elders. *Annals of Internal Medicine, 135* (2), 244–251.

Battelle Memorial Institute, JIL Information Systems. (1998). *An overview of the scientific literature concerning fatigue, sleep, and the circadian cycle*. Prepared for the Office of the Chief Scientific and Technical Advisor for Human Factors. http://cf.alpa.org/internet/projects/ftdt/backgr/batelle.htm.

Beck, L., Morrow, B., Lipscomb, L. E., Johnson, C. H., Gaffield, M. E., Rogers, et al. (2002). Prevalence of selected maternal behaviors and experiences. Pregnancy Risk Assessment Monitoring System (PRAMS), 1999. *MMWR Surveillance Summary, 51*(2), 1–27.

Belar, C. D. (2004). The future of education and training in academic health centers. *Journal of Clinical Psychology in Medical Settings, 11*(2), 77–82.

Berkelman, R. (2004). Public health interactions with the public: Can quality be assured? "This call may be monitored for quality assurance purposes." *Journal of Public Health Policy, 25*(1), 78–84.

Berman, S. (2000). The AMA clinical quality improvement forum on addressing patient safety. *Joint Commission Journal on Quality Improvement, 26*(7), 428–433.

Berwick, D. (2002). A user's guide to the IOM's Quality Chasm report. *Health Affairs, 21*(3), 80–90.

Berwick, D. M. (2002). A user's manual for the IOM's "Quality Chasm report": Patients' experiences should be the fundamental source of the definition of "quality." *Health Affairs (Millwood), 21*(1), 80–90.

Betacourt, J. (2004). *Unequal Treatment.* Presentation at University of Cincinnati College of Medicine, December 7.

Bodenheimer, T., Lorig, K., Holman, H., & Grumbach, K. (2002). Patient self-management of chronic disease in primary care. *Journal American Medical Assocation, 288*(19), 2469–2475.

Bolton, L. B., & Goodenough, A. (2003). A magnet nursing service approach to nursing's role in quality improvement. *Nursing Administration Quarterly, 27*(4), 344–354.

Bower, F., & McCullough, C. (2000). Restraint use in acute care settings. *Journal of Nursing Administration, 30*(12), 592–598.

Brennan, T., Leape, L., Laird, N., Hebert, L., Localio, A. R., Lawthers, A. G., et al. (1991). Incidence of adverse events and negligence in hospitalized patients: Results of the Harvard medical practice study I. *New England Journal of Medicine, 324*, 370–76.

Brooten, D., Youngblut, J., Kutcher, J., & Bobo, C. (2004). Quality and the nursing workforce: APNs, patient outcomes, and healthcare costs. *Nursing Outlook, 52*(1), 45–52.

Broyles, R., Tyson, J. E., Heyne, E. T., Heyne, R. J., Hickman, J. F., Swint, et al. (2000). Comprehensive follow-up care and life-threatening illnesses among high-risk infants: A randomized controlled trial. *Journal American Medical Association, 284*(16), 2070–2076.

Buerhaus, P., Staiger, D., & Auerbach, D. (2003). Is the current shortage of hospital nurses ending? *Health Affairs, 22*(6), 191–198.

Bukunt, S., Hunter, C., Perkins, S., Russell, D., & Domanico, L. (2005). El Camino Hospital: Using health information technology to promote patient safety. *Joint Commission Journal on Quality and Patient Safety, 31*(10), 561–565.

Bullen, B. (2002). The way across the chasm. IOM reports help providers, government navigate toward higher-quality care. *Modern Healthcare, 32*(46), 30.

Burt, C. W., & Hing, E. (2005). Use of computerized clinical support systems in medical settings: United States, 2001–03. *Advances in Data, 2*(353), 1–8.

Caldwell, C. (2001). Key themes of the analysis of the IOM reports. *Frontiers of Health Services Management, 18*(1), 41–46, 51–52.

Centers for Disease Control and Prevention (CDC). (2002). Syndemics overview: What procedures are available for planning and evaluating initiatives to prevent syndemics? The National Center for Chronic Disease Prevention and Health Promotion Syndemics Prevention Network. http://www.cdc.gov/syndemics/overview-planeval.htm.

Chapman, T. (2004). Restring the safety net. Incremental changes aren't enough; a new system of care is needed. *Modern Healthcare, 34*(25), 22.

Chassin, M., Galvin, R., & the National Roundtable on Healthcare Quality. (1998). The urgent need to improve healthcare. *Journal American Medical Association, 280*, 1000–1005.

Cho, S. (2001). Nurse staffing and adverse patient outcomes: A systems approach. *Nursing Outlook, 49*, 78–85.

Cina, J., Baroletti, S., Churchill, W., Hayes, J., Messinger, C., Mogan-McCarthy, P., et al. (2004). Interdisciplinary education program for nurses and pharmacists. *American Journal of Health-System Pharmacy, 61*(21), 2294–2296.

Clark, S., & Connolly, C. (2004). Nurse education and patient outcomes: A commentary. *Policy, Politics, & Nursing Practice, 5*(1), 12–20.

Cobb, D. (2004). Improving patient safety—how can information technology help? *AORN Journal, 80*(2), 295–296, 298, 301–302.

Coffman, J., Seago, J., & Spetz, J. (2002). Minimum nurse-to-patient ratios in acute care hospitals in California. *Health Affairs, 21*(5), 53–64.

Cook, M. J., & Leathard, H. L. (2004). Learning for clinical leadership. *Journals of Nursing Management, 12*(6), 436–444.

Cooper, M. (2000). Towards a model of safety culture. *Safety Science, 36*, 111–36.

Cowen, M. J. (2004). Hallmarks of quality: Generating and using knowledge. *Communicating Nursing Research, 37*(1), 3–12.

Cringles, M. (2002). Developing an integrated care pathway to manage cancer pain across primary, secondary, and tertiary care. *Internal Journal of Palliative Nursing, 8*(5), 247–255.

Croke, E., & Mayberry, A. (2001). Physical restraint guidelines and care standards for use in nonpsychiatric acute care settings. *Journal of Legal Nurse Consulting, 12*(1), 3–7.

Curtin, L. (2001). Healing healthcare's organizational culture. *Seminars for Nurse Managers, 9*(4), 218–227.

Czaplinski, C., & Diers, D. (1998). The effect of staff nursing on length of stay and mortality. *Medical Care, 36*, 1626–1638.

Davidson, P. L., Andersen, R. M., Wyn, R., & Brown, E.R. (2004). A framework for evaluating safety-net and other community-level factors on access for low-income populations. *Inquiry, 41*(1), 21–38.

Detmer, D. E. (2001). A new health system and its quality agenda. *Frontiers of Health Service Management, 18*(1), 3–30.

Devers, K., Pham, H., & Liu, G. (2004). What is driving hospitals' patient-safety efforts? *Health Affairs, 23*(2), 103–115.

Dinges, D., Graeber, R. C., Rosekind, M. R., Samuel, A., & Wegmann, H. M. (1996). *Principles and guidelines for duty and rest scheduling in commercial aviation*. NASA Technical Memorandum 110404. Moffett Field, CA: National Aeronautics and Space Administration, Ames Research Center.

Dovidio, J., Brigham, J. C., Johnson, B. T., & Gaertner, S. L. (1996). Stereotyping, prejudice, and discrimination: Another look. In N. Macrae, C. Stangor, & M. Hewstone (Eds.), *Stereotypes and stereotying* (pp. 276–319). New York: Guilford.

Dutton, N., Gajewski, B., Taunton, R., & Moore, J. (2004). Nurse staffing and patient falls on acute care hospital units. *Nursing Outlook, 52*(1), 53–59.

Dyck, M. J. (2005). Evidence-based administrative guidelines: Quality improvement in nursing homes. *Journal of Gerontology Nursing, 31*(2), 4–10.

Elder-Van Hook, J. (2004). *Building a national agenda for simulation-based medical education.* Washington, DC: Advanced Initiatives in Medical Simulation.

Fairbrother, G., Kuttner, H., Miller, W., Hogan, R., McPhillips, H., Johnson, K. A., et al. (2000). Findings from case studies of state and local immunization programs. *American Journal of Preventive Medicine, 19*(3 Suppl), 54–77.

Fawcett, S., Francisco, V. T., Hyra, D., Paine-Andrews, A., Schultz, J. A., Russos, S., et al. (2000). Building healthy communities. In A. Tarlov & R. St. Peter (Eds.), *The society and population health reader: A state and community perspective* (pp. 75–93). New York: The New Press.

Feifer, C., & Ornstein, S. (2004). Strategies for increasing adherence to clinical guidelines and improving patient outcomes in small primary care practices. *Joint Commission Journal on Quality and Safety, 30*(8), 431–441.

Fleming, B., Silver, A., Ocepek-Welikson, K., & Keller, D. (2004). The relationship between organizational systems and clinical quality in diabetes care. *American Journal of Managed Care, 10*(12), 934–944.

Ford, E. W., Duncan, W. J., & Ginter, P. M. (2005). Health departments' implementation of public health's core functions: An assessment of health impacts. *Public Health, 119*(1), 11–21.

Fried, T., Bradley, E., Towle, V., & Allore, H. (2002). Understanding the treatment preferences of seriously ill patients. *New England Journal of Medicine, 346*(14), 1061–1066.

Gandhi, T. K. (2005). Fumbled handoffs: One dropped ball after another. *Annals of Internal Medicine, 142*(5), 352–358.

Gard, C. L., Flannigan, P. N., & Cluskey, M. (2004). Program evaluation: An ongoing systematic process. *Nursing Educational Perspectives, 25*(4), 176–179.

Gebbie, K., & Merrill, J. (2002). Public health worker competencies for emergency response. *Journal of Public Health Management & Practice, 8*(3), 73–81.

Gelinas, L. S., & Loh, D. Y. (2004). The effect of workforce issues on patient safety. *Nursing Econonics, 22*(5), 266–272, 279.

Gerteis, M., Edgman-Levetan, S., & Daley, J. (1993). *Through the patient's eyes. Understanding and promoting patient-centered care.* San Francisco, CA: Jossey-Bass.

Glasgow, R., Orleans, C., & Wagner, E. (2001). Does the chronic care model serve also as a template for improving prevention? *Milbank Quarterly, 79*(4), *iv–v*, 579–612.

Grissinger, M. C., Globus, N. J., & Fricker, M. P., Jr. (2003). The role of managed care pharmacy in reducing medication errors. *Journal of Managed Care Pharmacy, 9*(1), 62–65.

Grissinger, M. C., & Kelly, K. (2005). Reducing the risk of medication errors in women. *Journal of Women's Health (Larchmont), 14*(1), 61–67.

Hatcher, I., Sullivan, M., Hutchinson, J., Thurman, S., & Gaffney, F. A. (2004). An intravenous medication safety system: Preventing high-risk medication errors at the point of care. *Journal of Nursing Administration, 34*(10), 437–439.

Health Resources and Services Administration, Bureau of Health Professions, National Center for Health Workforce Analysis. (2004). *Projected supply, demand, and shortages of registered nurses: 2000-2020.* http://bhpr.hrsa.gov/healthworkforce/reports/rnproject/default.htm.

Healthcare errors report sparks major debate. (2000). *The American Nurse* (January/February), 8.

Helmreich, R. (2000). On error management: Lessons from aviation. *British Medical Journal, 320,* 781–785.

Hendrich, A. (2003). *Evidence-based design on nursing workspace in hospitals.* Report Commissioned by the IOM Committee on the Work Environment for Nurses and Patient Safety.

Hoffman, C., Rice, D., & Sung, H. (1996). Persons with chronic conditions: Their prevalence and costs. *Journal American Medical Association, 276*(18), 1473–1479.

Hogan, D. L., & Logan, J. (2004). The Ottawa model of research use: A guide to clinical innovation in the NICU. *Clinical Nurse Specialist, 18*(5), 255–261.

Horak, B. J., Welton, W., & Shortell, S. (2004). Crossing the quality chasm: Implications for health services administration education. *Journal of Health Administration Education, 21*(1), 15–38.

Horbar, J. D., Carpenter, J. H., Buzas J., Soll, R. F., Suresh, G., Bracken, M. B., Leviton, L. C., Plsek, P. E., & Sinclair, J. C. (2004). Collaborative quality improvement to promote evidence-based surfactant for preterm infants: A cluster randomised trial. *British Medical Journal, 329*(7473), 1004–1010.

Humphreys, J., Martin, H., Roberts, B., & Ferretti, C. (2004). Strengthening an academic nursing center through partnership. *Nursing Outlook, 52*(4), 197–202.

Hundert, E., Hafferty, F., & Christakis, D. (1996). Characteristics of the informal curriculum and trainees' ethical choices. *Academic Medicine, 71*(6), 624–642.

Institute of Medicine (IOM). (1995). Assessing the social and behavioral science base for HIV/AIDS prevention and intervention. Workshop summary and background papers. Washington, DC: National Academies Press.

Institute of Medicine (IOM). (1996). Wunderlich, G., Sloan, F., & Davis, C. (Eds.). *Nursing staffing in hospitals and nursing homes: Is it adequate?* Washington, DC: National Academies Press.

Institute of Medicine (IOM). (2000). *America's healthcare safety net: Intact but endangered.* Washington, DC: National Academies Press.

Institute of Medicine (IOM). (2004). *Insuring America's health: Principles and recommendations.* Washington, DC: National Academies Press.

James, N., Burrage, J., & Smith, B. (2003). Scientific integrity: a review of the Institute of Medicine's (IOM) reports. *Nursing Outlook, 51*(5), 239–241.

Jech, A. (2001). The next step in preventing med errors. *RN, 64*(4), 46–49.

Jencks, S. F. (2000). Clinical performance measurement: A hard sell. *Journal American Medical Association, 283*(15), 2015–2016.

Jennings, B., & McClure, M. (2004). Strategies to advance healthcare quality. *Nursing Outlook, 52*(1), 17–22.

Jha, A., Duncan, B., & Bates, D. (2001). Fatigue, sleepiness, and medical errors. In K. Shojania, B. Duncan, K. McDonald, & R. Wachter (Eds.), *Making healthcare safer: A critical analysis of patient safety practices.* Agency for Healthcare Research & Quality (AHRQ) Publication No. 01-E058. Rockville, MD: AHRQ.

Johnson, T., Currie, G., Keill, P., Corwin, S. J., Pardes, H., & Cooper, M. R. (2005). NewYork-Presbyterian Hospital: Translating innovation into practice. *Joint Commission Journal on Quality and Patient Safety, 31*(10), 554–560.

Joint Commission on Accreditation of Healthcare Organizations (JCAHO). (2002). *Healthcare at the crossroads. Strategies for addressing the evolving nursing crisis.* Oakbrook Terrace, IL: JCAHO.

Jones, B. (2002). Nurses and the code of silence. In M. D. Rosenthal and K. M. Sutcliffe (Eds.), *Medical error: What do we know? What do we do?* San Francisco, CA: Jossey-Bass.

Jones, M. (2001). Medical errors. *Journal of Legal Nurse Consultants, 12*(3), 16–19.

Kaplan, S., & Greenfield, S. (2004). The patient's role in reducing disparities. *Annals of Internal Medicine, 141*(3), 222–223.

Karch, A., & Karch, F. (2001). Take part in the solution. *American Journal of Nursing, 101*(10), 25.

Kaushal, R., Barker, K., & Bates, D. (2001). How can information technology improve patient safety and reduce medication errors in children's safety and reduce medication errors in children's healthcare? *Archives of Pediatric Adolescent Medicine, 155*(9), 1002–1007.

Kerfoot, K. (2004). Attending, questioning, and quality. *Nursing Economics, 22*(5), 282–284.

Kimball, B., & O'Neil, E. (2002). *Healthcare's human crisis: The American nursing shortage.* Princeton, NJ: The Robert Wood Johnson Foundation.

Kinnaman, M. L., & Bleich, M. R. (2004). Collaboration: Aligning resources to create and sustain partnerships. *Journal of Professional Nursing, 20*(5), 310–322.

Kizer, K. (1999). *Veterans Hospital Administration's (VHA's) patient safety improvement initiative.* Presentation to the National Health Policy Forum, May 14, Washington, DC.

Knos, S., & Gharrity, J. (2004). Creating a center for nursing excellence. *Journal of Nursing Administration Systems (JONAS) Healthcare, Law, Ethics, and Regulations, 6*(2), 44–53.

Kolarik, R., Arnold, R., Fischer, G., & Hanusa, B. (2002). Advance care planning. *Journal of General Internal Medicine, 17*(8), 618–624.

Kovner, C. (2001). The impact of staffing and the organization of work on patient outcomes and healthcare workers in healthcare organization. *Joint Commission Journal on Quality Improvement, 27*(9), 458–468.

Kovner, C., Mezey, M., & Harrington, C. (2000). Research priorities for staffing, case mix, and quality of care in U.S. nursing homes. *Journal of Nursing Scholarship, 32*(1), 77–80.

Lang, N., & Mitchell, P. (2004). Guest editorial: Quality as an enduring and encompassing concept. *Nursing Outlook, 52,* 1, 1–2.

Lang, N., Mitchell, P. H., Hinshaw, A. S., Jennings, B. M., Lamb, G .S., Mark, B. A, et al. (2004). Measuring and improving healthcare quality. *Medical Care, 42* (2), II-1–3.

LaVeist, T., Nickerson, K., & Bowie, J. (2000). Attitudes about racism, medical mistrust, and satisfaction with care among African American and white cardiac patients. *Medical Care Research and Review, 57* (Supplement 1), 146–161.

Lavizzo-Mourey, R., & Lumpkin, J. (2004). From unequal treatment to quality care. *Annals of Internal Medicine, 141*(3), 221.

Leape, L. (2002). Lucian Leape and healthcare errors. Interview by Pamela K. Scarrow and Susan V. White. *Journal for Healthcare Quality, 24*(3), 17–20.

Leatherman, S., & McCarthy, D. (2002). *Quality of health in the United States: A chartbook.* New York: The Commonwealth Fund.

Lichtig, L., Knauf, R., & Milholland, D. (1999). Some impacts of nursing on acute care hospital outcomes. *Journal of Nursing Administration, 29,* 23–33.

Lillie-Blanton, M., Brodie, M., Rowland, D., Altman, D., & McIntosh, M. (2000). Race, ethnicity, and the healthcare system: Public perceptions and experiences. *Medical Care Research and Review, 57*(1), 21–35.

Lober, W. G., Trigg, L., & Karras, B. (2004). Information system architectures for syndromeic surveillance. *Morbidity & Mortality Weekly Report (MMWR), 53* (Suppl), 203–208.

Longo, D. R., Hewett, J. E., Ge, B., & Schubert, S. (2005). The long road to patient safety: A status report on patient safety systems. *Journal American Medical Association, 294*(22), 2858–2865.

Maddox, P., Wakefield, M., & Bull, J. (2001). Patient safety and the need for professional and educational change. *Nursing Outlook, 49*(1), 8–13.

Manthous, C. A. (2005). Medical errors and quality of care in Connecticut hospitals: Grappling with the implications of the IOM reports. *Connecticut Medicine, 69*(1), 29–32.

Mantone, J. (2004). Welcome to the club. IOM reports on quality improvement of rural care. *Modern Healthcare, 34*(45), 14–15.

Maravilla, V., Graves, M. T., & Newcomer, R. (2005). Development of a standardized language for case management among high-risk elderly. *Lippincott's Case Management, 10*(1), 3–13.

Mark, B., Hughes, L., & Jones, C. (2004). The role of theory in improving patient safety and quality healthcare. *Nursing Outlook, 52*(1), 11–16.

Mark, B., Salyer, J., & Wan, T. (2003). Professional nursing practice: Impact on organization and patient outcomes. *Journal of Nursing Administration, 33*(4), 224–234.

Martin, P. A., Gustin, T. J., Uddin, D. E., & Risner, P. (2004). Organizational dimensions of hospital nursing practice: Longitudinal results. *Journal of Nursing Administration, 34*(12), 554–561.

Marx, D. (2001). Patient safety and the "just culture": A primer for healthcare executives. Funded by a grant from the National Heart, Lung, and Blood Institute, National Institutes of Health (Grant RO1 HL53772, Harold S. Kaplan, M.D., Principal Investigator). New York: Trustees of Columbia University.

Mattke, S., Needleman, J., Buerhaus, P., Stewart, M., & Zelevinsky, K. (2004). Evaluating the role of patient sample definitions for quality indicators sensitive to nurse staffing patterns. *Medical Care, 42* (2), II-21–33.

Mayo, A. M., & Duncan, D. (2004). Nurse perceptions of medication errors: What we need to know for patient safety. *Journal of Nursing Care Quality, 19*(3), 209–217.

McCain, G. (2004). Gaps and disparities in neonatal nursing care. *Neonatal Network, 23*(5), 7–8.

McCartt, A., Rohrbaugh, J., & Hammer, M. (2000). Factors associated with falling asleep at the wheel among long-distance truck drivers. *Accident Analysis and Prevention, 32*, 493–504.

McNeil, B. (2001). Shattuck lecture—Hidden barriers to improvement in the quality of care. *New England Journal of Medicine, 345*(22), 1612–1620.

McNiel, N. O., Mackey, T. A., & Sherwood, G. D. (2004). Quality and customer service aspects of faculty practice. *Nursing Outlook, 52*(4), 189–196.

Melnyk, B., & Fineout-Overholt, E. (Eds.). (2005). *Evidence-based practice in nursing and healthcare.* Philadelphia: Lippincott Williams & Wilkins.

Meretoja, R., Leino-Kilpi, H., & Kaira, A. M. (2004). Comparison of nurse competence in different hospital work environments. *Journal of Nursing Management, 12*(5), 329–336.

Mitchell, P., & Lang, N. (2004). Framing the problem of measuring and improving healthcare quality: Has the quality health outcomes model been useful? *Medical Care, 42*, 12–20.

Monarch, K. (2003). Magnet hospitals' powerful force for excellence. *Reflections on Nursing Leadership, 29*(4), 10–13, 44.

Montgomery, J. E., Irish, J. T., Wilson, I. B., Chang, H., Li, A. C., Rogers, W. H., & Safran, D. G. (2004). Primary care experiences of Medicare beneficiaries, 1998 to 2000. *Journal of General Internal Medicine, 19*(10), 1064–1065.

Moore, K., Lynn, M., McMillen, B., & Evans, S. (1999). Implementation of the ANA report card. *Journal of Nursing Administration, 29*(6), 48–54.

Mosocco, D. (2001). Data management using outcomes-based quality improvement. *Home Care Provider,* (12), 205–211.

Murray, M. (2001). Outcomes of concurrent utilization review. *Nursing Economics, 19*(1), 17–23.

Mustard, L. (2002). The culture of patient safety. *Journal of Nursing Administration's (JONA's) Healthcare Law, Ethics, and Regulation, 4*(4), 111–115.

National Institutes of Health (NIH). (2002). *State-of-the-Science Conference Statement.* State-of-the-Science Conference on Symptom Management in Cancer: Pain, Depression, and Fatigue. Washington, DC: NIH.

National League for Nursing. (2003). *Centers of excellence in nursing education*. New York: NLN. http://www.nln.org/Excellence/hallmarks_indicators.htm.

National Quality Forum. (2002). NQF Project Brief: Measuring serious, avoidable adverse events in hospital care. *National Forum for Healthcare Quality Measurement and Reporting.* Washington, DC: National Quality Forum.

Needleman, J., Buerhaus, P., Mattke, S., Stewart, M., & Zelevinski, K. (2002). Nurse-staffing levels and the quality of care in hospitals. *New England Journal of Medicine, 346*, 1715–1722.

O'May, F., & Buchan, J. (1999). Shared governance: A literature review. *International Journal of Nursing Studies, 36*, 281–300.

Ornstein, S., Jenkins, R. G., Nietert, P. J., Feifer, C., Roylance, L. F., Nemeth, L., et al. (2004). A multimethod quality improvement intervention to improve preventive cardiovascular care: A cluster randomized trial. *Annals of Internal Medicine, 141*(7), 523–532.

Pape, T. (2003). Evidence-based nursing practice: To infinity and beyond. *Journal of Continuing Education in Nursing, 34*(4), 154–161.

Pincus, T. (2004). Will racial and ethnic disparities in health be resolved primarily outside of standard medical care? *Annals of Internal Medicine, 141*(3), 224–225.

Potempa, K. M., & Tilden, V. (2004). Building high-impact science: The dean as innovator. *Journal of Nursing Education, 43*(11), 502–505.

Rantz, M., & Connolly, R. (2004). Measuring nursing care quality and using large data sets in nonacute care settings: State of the science. *Nursing Outlook, 52*(1), 23–27.

Raymond, B., & Dold, C. (2002). *Clinical information systems: Achieving the vision.* Oakland, CA: Kaiser Permanente for Health Policy.

Reason, J. (1990). *Human error*. Cambridge, UK: Cambridge University Press.

Ricketts, T. (2001). *Community capacity to improve population health: Defining community*. Draft report. Princeton, NJ: Robert Wood Johnson Foundation.

Robert Wood Johnson Foundation (RWJF). (2000). New survey shows language barriers causing many Spanish-speaking Latinos to skip care. Fact sheet presented at press briefing, December 12, 2001. Washington, DC: RWJF.

Rolland, P. (2004). Occurrence of dispensing errors and efforts to reduce medication errors at the Central Arkansas Veteran's Healthcare System. *Drug Safety, 27*(4), 271–282.

Rowell, P. (2001). Lessons learned while collecting ANA indicator data. The American Nurses Association responds. *Journal of Nursing Administration, 31*(3), 130–131.

Ruderman, M. (2000). Resource guide to concepts and methods for community-based and collaborative problem-solving. Women's and Children's Health Policy Center, Johns Hopkins University School of Public Health. http://www.med.jhu.edu/wchpc/pub/resrcd.PDF.

Russell, L., Gold, M., Seigel, J., Daniels, N., & Weinstein, M. (1996). *Quality first: Better healthcare for all Americans—final report to the President of the United States*. Washington, DC: U.S. Government Printing Office.

Ryan, J., Stone, R., & Raynor, C. (2004). Using large data sets in long-term care to measure and improve quality. *Nursing Outlook, 52*(1), 38–44.

Rycroft-Malone, J. (2004). The PARIHS framework—a framework for guiding the implementation of evidence-based practice. *Journal of Nursing Care Quality, 19*(4), 297–304.

Sackett, D. L., Rosenberg, W. M., Gray, J. A., Haynes, R. B., & Richardson, W. S. (1996). Evidence-based medicine: What it is and what it isn't. *British Medical Journal, 312*, 71–72.

Salimbene, S. (1999). Cultural competence: A priority for performance improvement action. *Journal of Nursing Administration, 13*(3), 23–35.

Schein, E. (1999). *The corporate culture survival guide*. San Francisco, CA: Jossey-Bass.

Schulman, K. A., & Kim, J. J. (2000). Medical errors: How the U.S. government is addressing the problem. *Current Controlled Trials in Cardiovascular Medicine, 1*, 25–27.

Scott, P. (2004). Commentary. The contribution of universities to the development of the nursing workforce and the quality of patient care. *Journal of Nursing Management, 12*(6), 393–396.

Shortell, S., Gillies, R., & Anderson, D. (2000). *Remaking healthcare in America* (2nd ed.). San Francisco, CA: Jossey-Bass.

Simpson, R. L. (2004). The softer side of technology: How IT helps nursing care. *Nursing Administration Quarterly, 28*(4), 302–305.

Sims, C. (2003). Increasing clinical satisfaction and financial performance through nurse-driven process improvement. *Journal of Nursing Administration, 33*(2), 68–75.

Shojania, K. G., Duncan., B. W., McDonald, K. M., & Wachter, R. M. (Eds.). (2002). Safe but sound: Patient safety meets evidence-based medicine. *Journal of American Medical Association, 288*(4), 508–513.

Shojania, K., Duncan, B., McDonald, K., & Wachter, R. (Eds.). (2001). *Making healthcare safer: A critical analysis of patient safety practice*. Evidence Report/Technology Assessment Number 43. Agency for Healthcare Research and Quality Publications No. 01-E058. Rockville, MD: AHRQ.

Smith, J., & Crawford, L. (2002). *Report of findings from the 2001 employers' survey*. NCSBN Research Brief 3. Chicago: National Council of State Boards of Nursing, Inc.

Stankovic, A. K. (2004). The laboratory is a key partner in assuring patient safety. *Clinics in Laboratory Medicine, 24*(4), 1023–1035.

Stanton, M. (2004). Hospital nurse staffing and quality of care. *Research in Action*, (14), March.

Stein, M., & Deese, D. (2004). Addressing the next decade of nursing challenges. *Nursing Economics, 22*(5), 273–279.

Stiehl, R. R. (2004). Quality assurance requirements for contract/agency nurses. *Journal of Nursing Administration Systems (JONAS) Healthcare Law, Ethics, & Regulations, 6*(3), 69–74.

Stryer, D., & Clancy, C. (2005). Patients' Safety. *British Medical Journal, 330*(7491), 553–554.

Stubbings, L., & Scott, J. M. (2004). NHS workforce issues: Implications for future practice. *Journal of Health Organizations Management, 18*(2–3), 179–194.

Study of Clinical Relevant Indicators for Pharmacologic Therapy (SCRIPT). (2005). SCRIPT Coalition for Quality in Medication Use. http://www.scriptproject.org/faq.html.

Swan, B., & Boruch, R. (2004). Quality of evidence: Usefulness in measuring the quality of healthcare. *Medical Care, 42* (2), II-12–20.

Taylor, N. T. (2005). The Magnet IC pull. *Nurse Manager, 36*(1), 36–43.

Texas Medical Foundation. (2002). Diabetes quality improvement project. http://www.tmf.org/diabetes/.

Trossman, S. (2004). Infection Control. *The American Nurse, 36*(1), 1, 9.

U.S. Department of Health and Human Services (DHHS). (2001). *Nurse staffing and patient outcomes in hospitals.* Washington, DC: DHHS.

Vahey, D., Swan, B., Lang, N., & Mitchell, P. (2004). Measuring and improving healthcare quality: Nursing's contributions to the state of science. *Nursing Outlook, 52,* 1, 6–10.

Van Ryn, M., & Burke, J. (2000). The effect of patient race and socio-economic disparities in medical care. *Medical Care, 40*(1), I-140–151.

Van-Griever, A., & Meijman, T. (1987). The impact of abnormal hours of work on various modes of information processing: A process model on human costs of performance. *Ergonomics, 30,* 1287–1299.

Vincent, C. (2003). Understanding and responding to adverse events. *New England Journal of Medicine, 348*(11), 1051–1056.

Von Korf, M., Gruman, J., Schaefer, J., Curry, S. J., & Wagner, E. H. (1997). Collaborative management of chronic illness. *Annals of Internal Medicine, 127*(12), 1097–1102.

Wagner, E., Austin, B., Davis, C., Hindmarsh, M., Schaefer, J., & Bonomi, A. (2001). Improving chronic illness care: Translating evidence into action. *Health Affairs, 20*(6), 64–78.

Wagner, E., Austin, B., & Von Korf, M. (1996a). Improving outcomes in chronic illness. *Managed Care Quarterly, 4*(2), 12–25.

Wagner, E., Austin, B., & Von Korf, M. (1996b). Organizing care for patients with chronic illness. *Milbank Quarterly, 74*(4), 511–542.

Wakefield, M., & Maddox, P. (2000). Patient quality and safety problems in the U.S. healthcare system: Challenges for nursing. *Nursing Economics, 18,* 58–62.

Weil, T. P. (2001). Commentary: Public disclosure in the health field: Is there a relevant option? *American Journal of Medical Quality, 16*(1), 23–33.

Weiner, J. (2002). Keeping health care quality on the policy agenda. Leonard David Institute (LDI) Health Policy Seminar Series. http://www.upenn.edu/ldi/panel.html.

West, E. (2000). Organizational sources of safety and danger: Sociological contributions to the study of adverse events. *Quality Healthcare, 9,* 120–126.

Whelton, P. (2002). Primary prevention of hypertension: Clinical and public health advisory form the national high blood pressure education program. *Journal American Medical Association, 288*(15), 1882–1888.

Wolf, Z. (2001). Understanding medication errors. *Nursing Spectrum (Metro Edition)*, (1), 29–34.

Woodhouse, L. D., Livingood, W. C., Holland, D., Luisi, N., & Nguyen, T. (2004). Integrating public health training and graduate medical education: Facilitating changes recommended in the IOM Report. Presentation, Washington, DC: American Public Health Association (APHA).

Yeh, S. H., Hsiao, C. Y., Ho, T. H., Chiang, M. C., Lin, L. W., Hsu, C. Y., et al. (2004). The effects of continuing education in restraint reduction on novice nurses in intensive care units. *Journal of Nursing Research, 12*(3), 246–256.

Yoder-Wise, P. (2004). Health professions education and you. *Journal of Continuing Education in Nursing, 35*(5), 195.

Young, D. (2003). Nation unprepared for microbial threats, IOM reports. *American Journal of Health-System Pharmacy, 60*(9), 863–864, 866.

## *Additional References: Evidence-Based Practice and Research*

This selection of books and journals will help you and your students to gain a broad grasp of the growing body of literature on evidence-based nursing practice and research. This is one of the five core competencies found in *Health Professions Education* (IOM, 2003b), which frames the strategies presented in Part 3.

Alderson, P. (2001). Prenatal screening, ethics and Down's syndrome: A literature review. *Nursing Ethics, 8*(4), 360–374.

Allen, M. P., Jacobs, S. K., Levy, J., Pierce, S., Pravikoff, D. S., & Tanner, A. (2005). Continuing education as a catalyst for inter-professional collaboration. *Medical Reference Services Quarterly, 24*(3), 93–102.

Arnold, J. L. (2005). Risk and risk assessment in health emergency management. *Prehospital and Disaster Medicine, 20*(3), 143–154.

Atkins, D., Fink, K., & Slutsky, J. (2005). Better information for better healthcare: The evidence-based practice center program and the Agency for Healthcare Research and Quality. *Annals of Internal Medicine, 142*(12), 1035–1041.

Baldwin, C., & Fineout-Overholt, E. (2005). Evidence-based practice as holistic nursing research. *Beginnings, 25*(3), 16.

Bassand, J. P., Priori, S., & Tendera, M. (2005). Evidence-based vs. "impressionist" medicine: How best to implement guidelines. *European Heart Journal, 26*(12), 1155–1158.

Beech, I. (2005). Deconstructing evidence-based practice. *Journal of Psychiatric and Mental Health Nursing, 12*(4), 508–09.

Bellomo, R., Honore, P. M., Matson, J., Ronco, C., & Winchester, J. (2005). Extracorporeal blood treatment (EBT) methods in SIRS/Sepsis. *International Journal of Artificial Organs, 28*(5), 450–458.

Bernstein Ratner, N. (2005). Evidence-based practice in stuttering: Some questions to consider. *Journal of Fluency Disorders.*

Billi, J. E., Montgomery, W., Nolan, J., & Nadkarni, V. (2005). Guidelines for cardiopulmonary resuscitation. *Journal American Medical Association, 293*(22), 2713–2714.

Blatt, S. J., & Zuroff, D.C. (2005). Empirical evaluation of the assumptions in identifying evidence-based treatments in mental health. *Clinical Psychology Review, 25*(4), 459–486.

Bolukbas, C., Bolukbas, F. F., Kendir, T., Dalay, R. A., Akbayir, N., Sokmen, M. H., et al. (2005). Clinical presentation of abdominal tuberculosis in HIV seronegative adults. *BMC Gastroenterology, 5*(1), 21.

Briggs, A. (2005). Evidence-based practice is not the whole answer. *Australian Journal of Physiotherapy, 51*(2), 132–133.

Brosnan, C. A., Upchurch, S. L., Meininger, J. C., Hester, L. E., Johnson, G., & Eissa, M. A. (2005). Student nurses participate in public health research and practice through a school-based screening program. *Public Health Nursing, 22*(3), 260–266.

Brown, R. T., Amler, R. W., Freeman, W. S., Perrin, J. M., Stein, M. T., Feldman, H. M., et al. (2005). Treatment of attention-deficit/hyperactivity disorder: Overview of the evidence. *Pediatrics, 115*(6), 749–757.

Brown, S. (1999). *Knowledge for healthcare practice: A guide to using research evidence.* Philadelphia: Saunders.

Burkiewicz, J. S., & Zgarrick, D. P. (2005). Evidence-based practice by pharmacists: Utilization and barriers. *Annals of Pharmacotherapy, 39*(7), 1214–1219.

Carr, D. B., Reines, H. D., Schaffer, J., Polomano, R. C., & Lande, S. (2005). The impact of technology on the analgesic gap and quality of acute pain management. *Regional Anesthesia and Pain Medicine, 30*(3), 286–291.

Casey, A. (2005). Accessing research. *Paediatric Nursing, 17*(4), 3.

Cayley, W. E., Jr. (2005). Evidence-based medicine for medical students: Introducing EBM in a primary care rotation. *Wisconsin Medical Journal, 104*(3), 34–37.

Chinman, M., Hannah, G., Wandersman, A., Ebener, P., Hunter, S. B., Imm, P., et al. (2005). Developing a community science research agenda for building community capacity for effective preventive interventions. *American Journal of Community Psychology, 35*(3–4), 143–157.

Choi, B. C., Pang, T., Lin, V., Puska, P., Sherman, G., Goddard, M., et al. (2005). Can scientists and policy makers work together? *Journal of Epidemiology and Community Health, 59*(8), 632–637.

Chou, R., & Helfand, M. (2005). Challenges in systematic reviews that assess treatment harms. *Annals of Internal Medicine, 142*(12 Pt 2), 1090–1099.

Chou, R., Huffman, L. H., Fu, R., Smits, A. K., & Korthuis, P. T. (2005). Screening for HIV: A review of the evidence for the U.S. Preventive Services Task Force. *Annals of Internal Medicine, 143*(1), 55–73.

Chou, R., Smits, A. K., Huffman, L. H., Fu, R., & Korthuis, P. T. (2005). Prenatal screening for HIV: A review of the evidence for the U.S. Preventive Services Task Force. *Annals of Internal Medicine, 143*(1), 38–54.

Coster, W. (2005). International conference on evidence-based practice: A collaborative effort of the American Occupational Therapy Association, the American Occupational Therapy Foundation, and the Agency for Healthcare Research and Quality. *American Journal of Occupational Therapy, 59*(3), 356–358.

Cross, H. (2005). Consensus methods: A bridge between clinical reasoning and clinical research? *International Journal of Leprosy and Other Mycobacterial Diseases, 73*(1), 28–32.

Cuthill, F. M., & Espie, C. A. (2005). Sensitivity and specificity of procedures for the differential diagnosis of epileptic and non-epileptic seizures: A systematic review. *Seizure, 14*(5), 293–303.

Dale, A. E. (2005). Evidence-based practice: Compatibility with nursing. *Nursing Standard, 19*(40), 48–53.

Dale, J. C. (2005). Critiquing research for use in practice. *Journal of Pediatric Healthcare, 19*(3), 183–186.

Davis, D. W. (2005). The integration of research and practice: The importance of examining the evidence. *Neonatal Network, 24*(3), 77–79.

Duffy, M. E. (2005). The Agency for Healthcare Research and Quality: A valuable resource for evidence-based practice. *Clinical Nurse Specialist, 19*(3), 117–120.

Duke, G., Santamaria, J., Shann, E., & Stow, P. (2005). Outcome-based clinical indicators for intensive care medicine. *Anaesthesia and Intensive Care, 33*(3), 303–310.

Fineout-Overholt, E., Levin, R. F., & Melnyk, B. M. (2004). Strategies for advancing evidence-based practice in clinical settings. *Journal of New York State Nurses Association, 35*(2), 28–32.

Flynn, L. (2005). The importance of work environment: Evidence-based strategies for enhancing nurse retention. *Home Healthcare Nurse, 23*(6), 366–371.

Foxcroft, D., & Cole, N. (2005). Organizational infrastructure to promote evidence-based nursing practice. *Cochrane Review*, May.

Friedland, D., Go, A., Davoren, J., Bent, S., Subak, L., & Mendolson, T. (1999). *Evidence-based medicine: A framework for clinical practice.* Stamford, CT: Appleton & Lange.

Ghosh, A. K., & Ghosh, K. (2005). Translating evidence-based information into effective risk communication: Current challenges and opportunities. *Journal of Laboratory and Clinical Medicine, 145*(4), 171–180.

Giedt, J. (2005). Evidence-based practice: Just what is it? *Prairie Rose, 74*(2), 21.

Glasgow, R. E., Magid, D. J., Beck, A., Ritzwoller, D., & Estabrooks, P. A. (2005). Practical clinical trials for translating research to practice: Design and measurement recommendations. *Medical Care, 43*(6), 551–557.

Harrison, M. B., Graham, I. D., Lorimer, K., Friedberg, E., Pierscianowski, T., & Brandys, T. (2005). Leg-ulcer care in the community, before and after implementation of an evidence-based service. *Canadian Medical Association Journal, 172*(11), 1447–1452.

Hassed, C. (2005). An integrative approach to asthma. *Australian Family Physician, 34*(7), 573–576.

Hertel, J. (2005). Research training for clinicians: The crucial link between evidence-based practice and third-party reimbursement. *Journal of Athletic Training, 40*(2), 69–70.

Killeen, M. B., & Barnfather, J. S. (2005). A successful teaching strategy for applying evidence-based practice. *Nurse Educator, 30*(3), 127–132.

Kleinpell, R., & Gawlinski, A. (2005). Assessing outcomes in advanced practice nursing: The use of quality indicators. *AACN Issues*, January.

Melnyk, B., & Finehout-Overholt, E. (2005). *Evidence-based practice in nursing and healthcare.* Philadelphia: Lippincott Williams & Wilkins.

Nolan, M. R. (2005). Reconciling tensions between research, evidence-based practice and user participation: Time for nursing to take the lead. *International Journal of Nursing Studies, 42*(5), 503–505.

Ohio Board of Nursing. (2005). Medication aide pilot program planning begins. *Momentum, 3*(4), 13–14.

Paramonczyk, A. (2005). Barriers to implementing research in clinical practice. *Canadian Nurse, 101*(3), 12–15.

Pierce, S. T. (2005). Integrating evidence-based practice into nursing curricula. In *Annual review of nursing education: Strategies for teaching, assessment, and program planning* (pp. 233–248). New York: Springer Publisher.

Porter O'Grady, Tim. (2004). *The Future of Leaders in the Nursing Profession.* Presentation to the annual meeting of the American Academy of Nursing. Washington, DC: J. W. Marriott.

Raina, P., O'Donnell, M., Rosenbaum, P., Brehaut, J., Walter, S. D., Russell, D., et al. (2005). The health and well-being of caregivers of children with cerebral palsy. *Pediatrics, 115*(6), 626–636.

Rosswurm, M. A., & Larabee, J. H. (1999). A model for change to evidence-based practice. *Image: The Journal of Nursing Scholarship, 31*, 317–322.

Sackett, D. L., Rosenberg, W. M. C., Gray, J. A. M., Haynes, R. B., & Richardson, W. S. (1996). Evidence-based medicine: What it is and what it isn't. *British Medical Journal, 312*, 71–72.

Sakala, C. (2005a). Current resources for evidence-based practice. *Journal of Obstetric, Gynecologic, and Neonatal Nursing, 34*(4), 500–503.

Sakala, C. (2005b). Current resources for evidence-based practice. *Journal of Midwifery and Womens Health, 50*(4), 354–356.

Salzman, C. (2005). The limited role of expert guidelines in teaching psychopharmacology. *Academic Psychiatry, 29*(2), 176–179.

Smith, S. C. (2005). Confused about evidence based nursing practice? *Insight, 30*(1), 6.

Steele, R. W. (2005). Chronic sinusitis in children. *Clinical Pediatrics (Phila), 44*(6), 465–471.

Stevens, K. R. (2005). *Essential competencies for evidence-based practice in nursing* (1st ed.). San Antonio, TX: The University of Texas Health Science Center at San Antonio.

Stevens, K., & Cassidy, V. (1999). *Evidence-based teaching.* Sudbury, MA: National League for Nursing.

Sudsawad, P. (2005). A conceptual framework to increase usability of outcome research for evidence-based practice. *American Journal of Occupational Therapy, 59*(3), 351–355.

Upton, D., & Upton, P. (2005). Nurses' attitudes to evidence-based practice: Impact of a national policy. *British Journal of Nursing, 14*(5), 284–288.

Wills, C. E. (2005). What really works in clinical practice? Becoming more evidence based. *Journal of Psychosocial Nursing and Mental Health Services, 43*(4), 8–9.

# Appendix A
# Recommendations from the President's Advisory Commission on Consumer Protection and Quality in the Healthcare Industry

The purpose of the healthcare system must be to continuously reduce the impact and burden of illness, injury, and disability, and to improve the health and functioning of the people of the United States.

## Initial Set of National Aims

- Reducing the underlying causes of illness, injury, and disability
- Expanding research on new treatments and evidence on effectiveness
- Ensuring the appropriate use of healthcare services
- Reducing healthcare errors
- Addressing oversupply and undersupply of healthcare resources
- Increasing patients' participation in their care

Measurable objectives need to be specified for each of these aims.

## Advancing Quality Measurement and Reporting

A core set of quality measures should be identified for standardized reporting by each sector of the healthcare industry. There should be a stable and predictable mechanism for reporting. Steps should be taken to ensure that comparative information on healthcare quality is valid, reliable, comprehensible, and widely available in the public domain.

## *Creating Public-Private Partnerships*

An advisory council for healthcare quality should be created in the public sector to provide ongoing national leadership in promoting and guiding continuous improvement of healthcare quality. It would track and report on the progress of achieving the national aims for improvement, undertake related quality measurement and reporting, and implement the Consumer Bill of Rights and Responsibilities. A forum for healthcare quality measurement and reporting should be created in the private sector to improve the effectiveness and efficiency of healthcare quality measurement and reporting. Widespread public availability of comparative information on quality care needs to be provided.

## *Encouraging Action by Group Purchasers*

Group purchasers, to the extent feasible, should provide their individual members with a choice of plans. State and federal governments should create further opportunities for small employers to participate in large purchasing pools that, to the extent feasible, make a commitment to individual choice of plans. All public and private group purchasers should use quality as a factor in selecting the plans they will offer to their individual members, employees, or beneficiaries. Group purchasers should implement strategies to stimulate ongoing improvements in healthcare quality.

## *Strengthening the Hand of Consumers*

Widespread and ongoing consumer education should be developed to deliver accurate and reliable information and encourage consumers to consider information on quality when choosing health plans, providers, and treatments. Some consumers will require assistance in making these choices. Further research should be conducted addressing the use of consumer information.

## *Focusing on Vulnerable Populations*

Additional investment should be provided for developing, evaluating, and supporting effective healthcare delivery models designed to meet the specific needs of vulnerable populations.

## *Promoting Accountability*

The Consumer Bill of Rights and Responsibility should be included in private and public sector contractual and oversight requirements.

## *Reducing Errors and Increasing Safety in Health Care*

Interested parties should work together to develop a healthcare error reporting system to identify errors and prevent their recurrence.

## *Fostering Evidence-Based Practice and Innovation*

Federal funding for healthcare research, including basic, clinical, prevention, and health services research, should be increased and the necessary research infrastructure supported. Collaborative arrangements between researchers and private and public sectors should be developed. Research should target those areas where the greatest improvements in health and functional status of population can occur and where gaps in knowledge exist.

## *Adapting Organizations for Change*

Healthcare organizations should provide strong leadership to confront quality challenges and pursue aims for improvement. They should commit to reducing errors and increasing safety. Organizations need to develop long-term relationships with all stakeholders.

## *Engaging the Healthcare Workforce*

The training of physicians, nurses, and other healthcare workers must change to meet the demands of a changing healthcare industry. Minimum standards for education, training, and supervision of unlicensed paraprofessionals should be established. Steps should be taken to improve the diversity and the cultural competence of the healthcare workforce. Healthcare workers must be encouraged to identify and report clinical errors and instances of improper or dangerous care. Action must be taken to reduce the unacceptably high rate of injury in the healthcare workforce. Efforts must be taken to address the serious morale problems that exist among healthcare workers in many sectors of the industry. Further research should be conducted into how changes in the roles and responsibilities of healthcare workers are affecting quality.

## *Investing in Information Systems*

Purchasers of healthcare services should insist that providers and plans be able to produce quantitative evidence of quality as a means of encouraging investment in information systems.

*Source*: The President's Advisory Commission on Consumer Protection and Quality in the Healthcare Industry. (1999). *Quality first: Better health care for all Americans.* Washington, DC: U.S. Government Printing Office.

# *Appendix B*

# *Recommendations from* To Err Is Human

- Congress should create a Center of Patient Safety with the Agency for Healthcare Policy and Research. This Center should:
  - Set the national goals for patient safety, track progress in meeting these goals, and issue an annual report to the President and Congress on patient safety; and
  - Develop knowledge and understanding of errors in health care by developing a research agenda, funding Centers of Excellence, evaluating methods for identifying and preventing errors, and funding dissemination and communication activities to improve patient safety.
- A nationwide mandatory reporting system should be established that provides for the collection of standardized information by state governments about adverse events that result in death or serious harm. Reporting should initially be required of hospitals and eventually be required of other institutional and ambulatory care delivery settings. Congress should:
  - Designate the Forum for Healthcare Quality Measurement and Reporting as the entity responsible for promulgating and maintaining a core set of reporting standards to be used by states, including a nomenclature and taxonomy for reporting;
  - Require all healthcare organizations to report standardized information on a defined list of adverse events;
  - Provide funds and technical expertise for state governments to establish or adapt their current error reporting systems to collect the standardized information, analyze it, and conduct follow-up action as needed with healthcare organizations. Should a state choose not to implement the mandatory reporting system, the Department of Health and Human Services should be designated as the responsible entity; and designate the Center for Patient Safety to:
    1. convene states to share information and expertise, and to evaluate alternative approaches taken for implementing reporting programs, identify best practices for implementation, and assess the impact of state programs; and

    (2) receive and analyze aggregate reports from states to identify persistent safety issues that require more intensive analysis or a broader-based response (e.g., designing prototype systems or requesting a response by agencies, manufacturers, or others).

- The development of voluntary reporting efforts should be encouraged. The Center for Patient Safety should
  - Describe and disseminate information on external voluntary reporting programs to encourage greater participation in them and track the development of new reporting systems as they form;
  - Convene sponsors and users of external reporting systems to evaluate what works;
  - Periodically assess whether additional efforts are needed to address gaps in information, to improve patient safety, and to encourage healthcare organizations to participate in voluntary reporting programs; and
  - Fund and evaluate pilot projects for reporting systems, both within individual healthcare organizations and collaborative efforts among healthcare organizations.
- Congress should pass legislation to extend peer review protections to data related to patient safety and quality improvement that are collected and analyzed by healthcare organizations for internal use or shared with others solely for purposes of improving safety and quality.
- Performance standards and expectation for healthcare organization should focus greater attention on patient safety.
  - Regulators and accreditors should require healthcare organizations to implement meaningful patient safety programs with defined executive responsibility.
  - Public and private purchasers should provide incentives to healthcare organizations to demonstrate continuous improvement in patient safety.
- Performance standards and expectations for health professionals should focus greater attention on patient safety.
  - Health professional licensing bodies should
    (1) implement periodic re-examination and re-licensing of doctors, nurses, and other key providers, based on both competence and knowledge of safety practices; and
    (2) work with certifying and credentialing organizations to develop more effective methods to identify unsafe providers and take action.
  - Professional societies should make a visible commitment to patient safety by establishing a permanent committee dedicated to safety improvement. The committee should
    (1) develop a curriculum on patient safety and encourage its adoption into training and certification requirements;
    (2) disseminate information on patient safety to members through special sessions at annual conferences, journal articles, and editorials, newsletters, publications, and websites on regular basis;

(3) recognize patient safety considerations in practice guidelines and in standards related to the introduction and diffusion of new technologies, therapies, and drugs;
(4) work with the Center for Patient Safety to develop community-based, collaborative initiatives for error reporting and analysis and implementation of patient safety improvements; and
(5) collaborate with other professional societies and disciplines in a national summit on the professional's role in patient safety.

- The Food and Drug Administration (FDA) should increase attention to the safe use of drugs in both pre- and post-marketing processes through the following actions:
  - Develop and enforce standards for the design of drug packaging and labeling that will maximize safety in use;
  - Require pharmaceutical companies to test (using FDA-approved methods) proposed drug names to identify and remedy potential sound-alike and look-alike confusion with existing drug names; and
  - Work with physicians, pharmacists, consumers, and others to establish appropriate response to problems identified through post-marking surveillance, especially for concerns that are perceived to require immediate response to protect the safety of patients.
- Healthcare organizations and the professionals affiliated with them should make continually improved patient safety a declared and serious aim by establishing patient safety programs with defined executive responsibility. Patient safety programs should
  - Provide strong, clear, and visible attention to safety;
  - Implement non-punitive systems for reporting and analyzing errors in their organization;
  - Incorporate well-understood safety principles, such as standardizing and simplifying equipment, supplies, and processes; and
  - Establish interdisciplinary team training programs for providers that incorporate proven methods of team training, such as simulation.
- Healthcare organizations should implement proven medication safety practices.

*Source*: Institute of Medicine (IOM). (1999). *To err is human. Building a safer health system.* Washington, DC: The National Academies Press. Reprinted with permission.

# Appendix C

# *Recommendations from* Crossing the Quality Chasm

- All healthcare constituents, including policymakers, purchasers, regulators, health professionals, healthcare trustees and management, and consumers, should commit to a national statement of purpose for the healthcare systems as a whole and to a shared agenda of six aims for improvement that can raise the quality of care to unprecedented levels. [*This is related to the six aims or goals identified by the report. This has never been done, and it will not be easy to accomplish. It also requires an interdisciplinary solution to a multifaceted problem—again an approach never before attempted on a national scale. Nursing education needs to be part of the interdisciplinary solution as an active team member working collaboratively with other healthcare educations such as medicine, pharmacy, and allied health.*]
- Clinicians and patients, and the healthcare organizations that support care delivery, should adopt a new set of principles to guide the redesign of care processes. [*Identifying critical concerns will be important. Often clinicians, patients, and healthcare organizations do not agree, but consensus will be important for success.*]
- The Department of Health and Human Services (DHHS) should identify a set of priority conditions to focus initial efforts, provide resources to stimulate innovation, and initiate the change process. [*A later IOM report,* Priority Areas for National Action *(Greiner& Knebel, 2003), identifies these conditions.*]
- Healthcare organizations should design and implement more effective organizational support processes to make change in the delivery of care possible. [*Change is ever present, and healthcare organizations and their leaders and staff must learn more effective methods for coping with change.*]
- Purchasers, regulators, health professions, educational institutions-key stakeholders, and the DHHS should create an environment that fosters and rewards improvement by
  (1) creating an infrastructure to support evidence-based practice,
  (2) facilitating the use of information technology (IT),
  (3) aligning payment incentives, and

(4) preparing the workforce to better serve patients and their families in a world of expanding knowledge and rapid change.

[*There is no doubt that these are key issues. Through its web site, DHHS has provided some infrastructure to support evidence-based practice such as the work done by AHRQ, but more support is needed. As discussed in Part 1, the IOM report* Patient Safety *addresses some of the needs in IT and standards. Financial issues and reimbursement are also areas of deep concern.*]

*Source*: Institute of Medicine. (IOM). (2001). *Crossing the quality chasm*. Washington, DC: The National Academies Press. Reprinted with permission.

# Appendix D
# National Healthcare Quality Report Matrix

| Consumer Perspectives on Healthcare Needs | Components of Healthcare Quality | | | |
|---|---|---|---|---|
| | *Safety* | *Effectiveness* | *Patient Centeredness* | *Timeliness* |
| Staying Healthy | | | | |
| Getting Better | | | | |
| Living with Illness or Disability | | | | |
| Coping with the End of Life | | | | |

*Source*: Institute of Medicine (IOM). (2001). *Envisioning the National Healthcare Quality*. Washington, DC: National Academies Press, p. 61. Reprinted with permission.

# *Appendix E*

# *Recommendations from* Leadership by Example

- The federal government should assume a strong leadership position in driving the healthcare sector to improve the safety and quality of healthcare services provided to the approximately 100 million beneficiaries of the six major government healthcare programs. Given the leverage of the federal government, this leadership will result in improvements in the safety and quality of health care provided to all Americans.
- The federal government should take maximal advantage of its unique position as regulator, healthcare purchaser, healthcare providers and sponsor of applied health services research to set quality standards for the healthcare sectors. Specifically:
  - Regulatory processes should be used to establish clinical data reporting requirements applicable to all six major government healthcare programs.
  - All six major government healthcare programs should vigorously pursue purchasing strategies that encourage that adoption of best practices through the release of public-domain comparative quality data and the provision of financial and other rewards for providers that achieve high levels of quality.
  - Not only should healthcare delivery systems operated by the public programs continue to serve as laboratories for the development of innovative twenty-first-century care delivery models, but much greater emphasis should be placed on the dissemination of the findings and, in the case of information technology, the creation of public-domain products.
  - Applied health services research should be expanded and should emphasize the development of knowledge, tools, and strategies that can support quality enhancement in a wide variety of settings.
- Congress should direct the Secretaries of the Department of Health and Human Services, Department of Defense, and Department of Veterans Affairs to work together to establish standardized performance measures across the government programs, as well as public reporting requirements for clinicians, institutional providers, and health plans in each program. These requirements should be implemented for all six major government healthcare programs and

should be applied fairly and equitably across various financing and delivery options in those programs. The standardized measurement and reporting activities should replace the many performance measurement activities currently under way in the various government programs.

- The Quality Interagency Coordination Task Force (QuIC) should promulgate standardized sets of performance measures for five common health conditions in fiscal year (FY) 2003 and another 10 sets in FY 2004.
  - Each government healthcare program should pilot test the first set of measures between FY 2003 and FY 2005 in a limited number of sites. These pilot tests should include the collection of patient-level data and the public release of comparative performance reports.
  - All six government programs should prepare for full implementation of the 15-set performance measurement and reporting system by FY 2008. The government healthcare programs that provide services through the private sector (i.e., Medicare, Medicaid, SCHIP, and portions of DOD TRICARE) should inform participating providers that submission of the audited patient-level data necessary for performance measurement will be required for continued participation in FY 2007. The government healthcare programs that provide services directly (i.e., VHA, the remainder of DOD TRICARE, and HIS) should begin work immediately to ensure that they have the information technology capabilities to produce the necessary data.
- The Federal government should take steps immediately to encourage and facilitate the development of the information technology infrastructure that is critical to healthcare quality and safety enhancement, as well as to many of the nation's other priorities, such as bioterrorism surveillance, public health, and research. Specifically:
  - Congress should consider potential options to facilitate rapid development of a national health information infrastructure, including tax credits, subsidized loans, and grants.
  - Government healthcare programs that deliver services through the private sector (Medicare, Medicaid, SCHIP, and a portion of DOD TRICARE) should adopt both market-based and regulatory options to encourage investment in information technology. Such options might include enhanced or more rapid payments to providers capable of submitting computerized clinical data, a requirement for certain information technology capabilities as a condition of participation, and direct grants.
  - VHA, DOD, and HIS should continue implementing clinical and administrative information systems that enable the retrieval of clinical information across their programs and can communicate directly with each other. Whenever possible, the software and intellectual property developed by these three government programs should rely on web-based language and architecture and be made available in the public domain.

- Starting in FY 2008, each government healthcare program should make comparative quality reports and data available in the public domain. The programs should provide for access to these reports and data in ways that meet the needs of various users, provided that patient privacy is protected.
- The government healthcare programs, working with Agency for Health Research Quality (AHRQ), should establish a mechanism for pooling performance measurement data across programs in a data repository. Contributions of data from private-sector insurance programs should be encouraged provided such data meet certain standards for validity and reliability. Consumers, healthcare professionals, planners, purchasers, regulators, public health officials, researchers, and others should be afforded access to the repository provided that patient privacy is protected.
- The six government healthcare programs should work together to develop a comprehensive health services research agenda that will support the quality enhancement processes of all programs. The QuIC (or some similar interdepartmental structure with representation from each of the government healthcare programs and AHRQ) should be provided the authority and resources needed to carry out this responsibility. The agenda for FY 2003–2005 should support the following:
  - Establishment of core sets of standardized performance measures.
  - Ongoing evaluation of the impact of the use of standardized performance measurement and reporting by the six major government healthcare programs.
  - Development and evaluation of specific strategies that can be used to improve the federal government's capability to leverage the purchaser, regulator, and provider roles to enhance quality.
  - Monitoring of national progress in meeting the six national quality aims (safety, effectiveness, patient-centeredness, timeliness, efficiency, and equity).

*Source*: Institute of Medicine (IOM). (2003). *Leadership by example: Coordinating government roles in improving healthcare quality.* Washington, DC: National Academies Press.

# Appendix F
# *Recommendations from* The Future of the Public's Health

Healthcare providers responsible for assuring population health need to focus on the following areas of action and change (IOM, 2003a, p. 4):

- Adopting a population health approach that considers the multiple determinants of health;
- Strengthening the governmental public health infrastructure, which forms the backbone of the public health system;
- Building a new generation of intersectoral partnerships that also draw on the perspectives and resources of diverse communities and actively engage them in health action;
- Developing systems of accountability to assure the quality and availability of public health services;
- Making evidence the foundation of decision-making and the measure of success; and
- Enhancing and facilitating communication in the public health system (e.g., among all levels of the governmental public health infrastructure and between public health professionals and community members).

Each of these action areas has relevance to nursing education; baccalaureate level students need some appreciation of how these action areas might be implemented, and graduate students in community health need to be directly involved in activities related to these action areas.

## *Recommendations for Nursing*

Achieving improvement in public health requires an acknowledgement and understanding of trends that affect health. There have been and will continue to be major changes in demographics and population growth, for example, greater diversity, aging population, and disparities. Technology and scientific research are rapidly moving forward providing opportunities and challenges. Information technology (IT) is discussed in the body of this document, particularly its impact on healthcare delivery, quality, and safety. Utilization of IT in public health requires consideration of issues such as sharing of information across healthcare organizations, communicable disease data, and more current issues such as the fear of bioterrorism and how this information should be shared in a timely manner.

Globalization has also had an impact on health in the United States. Diversity is one result, but also travel and communication allows U.S. citizens to interact with and share knowledge with others. In addition, there is greater exchange of products, such as pharmaceuticals and food, all of which are positive, but also carry risks such as spread of diseases or contaminated food. Bioterrorism is a critical concern with major implications for public health, and with the movement of greater globalization there is a greater risk. This concern is also changing the way public health is viewed. Prior to September 11, many thought of public health as epidemics, immunizations, and traveler warnings. Since that time the view has been on preparedness, including natural disasters and how we as a nation can respond. It has broadened the definition of public health to include information sharing, knowledge applications, and information networks necessary to speed responses in case of any emergency. This experience has unfortunately pointed out holes in the existing system, including communication problems among agencies and nonexistent databases that "talk" to each other for the purposes of rapid response. Disaster planning and bioterrorism are now included in most nursing curricula. Material has been developed to assist schools of nursing in this effort. For example, the Centers for Disease Control & Prevention (CDC) has funded projects in public health preparedness. They offer curriculum modules free of charge so that bioterrorism contact can be used by healthcare organizations and health professionals' education. These can be found through the CDC Office of Workforce Policy and Planning and the Specialty Centers in Public Health Preparedness (S-CPHPs). The Bureau of Health Professions and Department of Health and Human Services Health Resources & Services Administration (BHP and HRSA) have also funded grants to create continuing education programs as well as enhance curricula. Two such grants were awarded in 2004 to the University of Illinois at Chicago. Information on these grants can be found at http://www.hrsa.gov/bioterrorism/cooperative/index.htm

*Source*: Institute of Medicine (IOM). (2003a). *The future of the public's health.* Washington, DC: National Academies Press.

# *Appendix* G

# *Recommendations from* Who Will Keep the Public Healthy?

"A public health professional is a person educated in public health or a related discipline who is employed to improve heath through a population focus" (IOM, 2003b, p. 4). The eight content areas that are important for today's and future public health professions and should be included in nursing curricula are:

- Informatics
- Genomics
- Communication
- Cultural competence
- Community-based participatory research
- Global health, policy, and law
- Public health ethics

These are in addition to the longstanding core components of public health:

- Epidemiology
- Biostatistics
- Environmental health
- Health services administration
- Social and behavioral science

Recommendations for Nursing

- Understanding of public health in the community, health promotion, and disease prevention.
- Undergraduate nursing programs prepare students to understand the ecological model of health, its determinants, and core competencies in population-focused practice. This level of education and awareness will require that public health agencies support clinical experiences for nursing students.
- "Schools of nursing that offer master's degree programs in public health nursing should be encouraged to partner with schools of public health to ensure

that current thinking about public health is integrated into the nursing curricula content, and to facilitate development of interdisciplinary skills and capacities" (IOM, 2003b, p. 19). To do so effectively requires educational experiences through interdisciplinary work.

*Source*: Institute of Medicine (IOM). (2003). *Who will keep the public healthy?* Washington, DC: National Academies Press.

# Appendix H

# Recommendations from Keeping Patients Safe: Transforming the Work Environment for Nurses

- Healthcare organizations (HCOs) should acquire nurse leaders for all levels of management (e.g., at the organization-wide and patient care unit levels) who will:
  - articipate in executive decisions in the HCO.
  - Represent nursing staff to organization management and facilitate their mutual trust.
  - Achieve effective communication between nursing and other clinical leadership.
  - Facilitate input of direct-care nursing staff into operational decision-making and the design of work processes and work flow.
  - Be provided with organizational resources to support the acquisition, management, and dissemination to nursing staff of the knowledge needed to support their clinical decision-making and actions.
- Leaders of HCOs should take action to identify and minimize the potential adverse effects of their decisions on patient safety by:
  - Educating board members and senior, midlevel, and line managers about the link between management practices and safety.
  - Emphasizing safety to the same extent as productivity and financial goals in internal management planning and reports and in public reports to stakeholders.
- HCOs should employ management structures and processes throughout the organization that:
  - Provide ongoing vigilance in balancing efficiency and safety.
  - Demonstrate trust in workers and promote trust by workers.
  - Actively manage the process of change.
  - Engage workers in nonhierarchical decision-making and in the design of work processes and work flow.
  - Establish the organization as a "learning organization."

- Professional associations, philanthropic organizations, and other professional leaders in the healthcare industry should sponsor collaborative partnerships that incorporate multiple academic and other research-based organizations to support HCOs in the identification and adoption of evidence-based management practices.
- The U.S. Department of Health and Human Services (DHHS) should update regulations established in 1990 that specify minimum standards for registered and licensed nurse staffing in nursing homes. Updated minimum standards should:
  - Require the presence of at least one RN in the facility at all times.
  - Specify staffing levels that increase as the number of patients increase, and that are based on the findings and recommendations of the DHHS report to Congress, Appropriateness of Minimum Nurse Staffing Ratios in Nursing Homes—Phase II Final Report.
  - Address staffing levels for nurse assistants, who provide the majority of patient care.
- Hospitals and nursing homes should employ nurse staffing practices that identify needed nurse staffing for each patient care unit per shift. These practices should:
  - Incorporate estimates of patient volume that count admissions, discharges, and "less than full-day" patients in addition to a census of patients at a point in time.
  - Involve direct-care nursing staff in determining and evaluating the approaches used to determine appropriate unit staffing levels for each shift.
  - Provide for staffing "elasticity" or "slack" in each shift's scheduling to accommodate unpredicted variations in patient volume and acuity and their effect on workload. Methods used to provide slack should give preference to scheduling excess staff and creating cross-trained float pools in the HCO. Use of nurses from external agencies should be avoided.
- Hospitals and nursing homes should perform ongoing evaluation of the effectiveness of their nurse staffing practices with respect to patient safety, and increase internal oversight of their staffing methods, levels, and effects on patient safety whenever staffing falls below the following levels for a 24-hour day:
  - In hospital ICUs: one licensed nurse for every two patients (12 hours of licensed nursing staff per patient day).
  - In nursing homes, for long-term residents: one RN for every 32 patients (0.75 hours per resident day), one licensed nurse for every 18 patients (1.3 hours per resident day), and one nurse assistant for every 8.5 patients (2.8 hours per resident day).
- DHHS should implement a nationwide, publicly accessible system for collecting and managing valid and reliable staffing and turnover data from hospitals and nursing homes. Information on individual hospital and nursing home staffing at the level of individual nursing units and the facility in the aggregate should be disclosed routinely to the public.

    - Federal and state nursing home report cards should include standardized, case-mix-adjusted information on the average hours per patient day of RN, licensed, and nurse assistant care provided to residents and a comparison with federal and state standards.
    - During the next three years, public and private sponsors of the new hospital report card to be located on the federal government website should undertake an initiative—in collaboration with experts in acute hospital care, nurse staffing, and consumer information—to develop, test, and implement measures of hospital nurse staffing levels for the public.
- HCOs should dedicate funds equal to a defined percentage of nursing payroll to support nursing staff in their ongoing acquisition and maintenance of knowledge and skills. These resources should be sufficient for and used to implement policies and practices that:
    - Assign experienced nursing staff to precept nurses newly practicing in a clinical area to address gaps in knowledge or skills.
    - Annually ensure that each licensed nurse and nurse assistant has an individualized plan and resources for educational development in health care.
    - Provide education and training of staff as new technology or changes in the workplace are introduced.
    - Provide decision support technology to actively involve direct-care nursing staff in point-of-care learning.
    - Disseminate to individual staff members organizational learning as captured in clinical tools, algorithms, and pathways.
- To reduce error-producing fatigue, state regulatory bodies should prohibit nursing staff from providing patient care in any combination of scheduled shifts, mandatory overtime, or voluntary overtime in excess of 12 hours in any given 24-hour period and in excess of 60 hours per seven-day period. To this end:
    - HCOs and labor organizations representing nursing staff should establish policies and practices designed to prevent nurses who provide direct patient care from working longer than 12 hours in a 24-hour period and in excess of 60 hours per seven-day period.
    - Schools of nursing, state boards of nursing, and HCOs should educate nurses about the threats of patient safety caused by fatigue.
- HCOs should provide nursing leadership with resources that enable them to design the nursing work environment and care processes to reduce errors. These efforts must directly involve direct-care nurses throughout all phases of work design and should concentrate on errors associated with:
    - Surveillance of patient health status.
    - Patient transfers and other patient hand-offs.
    - Complex patient care processes
    - Non-value-added activities performed by nurses, such as locating and obtaining supplies, looking for personnel, completing redundant or unnecessary documentation, and compensating for poor communication systems.

- HCOs should address handwashing and medication administration among their first work design initiatives.
- Regulators, leaders in health care, and experts in nursing, law, informatics, and related disciplines should jointly convene to formulate strategies for safely reducing the burden associated with patient and work-related documentation.
- HCO boards of directors, managerial leadership, and labor partners should create and sustain cultures of safety by implementing the recommendations presented previously and by:
  - Specifying short- and long-term safety objectives.
  - Continuously reviewing success in meeting these objectives and providing feedback at all levels.
  - Conducting an annual, confidential survey of nursing and other healthcare workers to assess the extent to which a culture of safety exists.
  - Instituting a de-identified, fair, and just reporting system for errors and near misses.
  - Engaging in ongoing employee training in error detection, analysis, and reduction.
  - Implementing procedures for analyzing errors and providing feedback to direct-care workers.
  - Instituting rewards and incentives for error reduction.
- The National Council of State Boards of Nursing, in consultation with patient safety experts and healthcare leaders, should undertake an initiative to design uniform processes across states for better distinguishing human errors from willful negligence and intentional misconduct, along with guidelines for their application by state boards of nursing and other state regulatory bodies with authority over nursing.
- Congress should pass legislation to extend peer review protections to data related to patient safety and quality improvement that are collected and analyzed by HCOs for internal use or shared with others solely for purposes of improving safety and quality.

*Source*: Institute of Medicine (IOM). (2004). *Keeping patients safe. Transforming the work environment of nurses*. Washington, DC: National Academies Press. Reprinted with permission.

# Appendix I
# Strategies and Recommendations from Health Professions Education: A Bridge to Quality

## "Strategies

1. Develop a common language and core competencies.

   *Vision:* Across health professions schools and practice environments, there is a shared definition of key terms and competencies for education healthcare professionals. While the roles of individual health professionals vary with respect to each of the competencies, these shared definitions transcend occupations and enable cross-disciplinary communication. They enable interdisciplinary groups to define and reach consensus around a core set of competencies for health professions education.

2. Integrate core competencies into oversight processes.

   *Vision:* There is consistency in approach and coordination across the various health professions oversight organizations—including accrediting, licensing, and certification bodies—as the result of a course on an agreed-on set of core competencies. This consistency allows for enhanced communication, integration, and synergy within and across oversight bodies and professions. As a result, educational programs are evaluated based on outcomes, and a clinician's competency is assessed upon entry into practice and regularly throughout their career.

3. Motivate and support leaders and monitor profess of reform effort.

   *Vision:* An interdisciplinary group of education leaders—from practice environments and academic and continuing education settings, including students—works to create a shared mission for health professions education that relates to but is larger than the five competencies. This reform-minded group monitors progress in integrating the competencies into health professions education, and provides a regular status report to the larger education and quality communities. The group also supports leadership training for education leaders, recognizes and rewards leaders who make a significant contribution to education reform, and continuously assesses changing skill needs for health professionals.

5. Develop evidence-based curricula and teaching approaches.

   *Vision:* A rich, readily available evidence base exists to make the case for teaching the five competencies to health professions students and clinicians, demonstrating the strong relationship between these competencies and enhanced quality outcomes for patients. This evidence base is integrated across all the health professions through links to profession-specific databases. In addition, those who instruct and mentor health professionals in both academic and continuing education settings have access to a well developed evidence base regarding the effectiveness of teaching methods and continuously updated best-practices database.

6. Develop faculty as teaching and learning experts.

   *Vision:* Faculty development programs exist at the national and regional levels for the array of health professional educators, focused on the overarching vision presented in this report. The programs, many of which are interdisciplinary, prepare faculty to convey the five competencies, as well as to adopt an evidence-based approach to education.

## *Recommendations*

1. Department of Health and Human Services (DHHS) and leading foundations should support an interdisciplinary effort focused on developing a common language, with the ultimate aim of achieving consensus across the health professions on a core set of competencies that includes patient-centered care, interdisciplinary teams, evidence-based practice, quality improvement, and informatics.

   *Implications for nursing education*: These five areas become the curricular framework for guiding didactic and clinical work. They relate to the program's terminal objectives.

2. DHHS should provide a forum and support for a series of meetings involving the spectrum of oversight organizations across and within the disciplines. Participants in these meetings would be charged with developing strategies for incorporating a core set of competencies into oversight activities, based on definitions shared across the professions. These meetings would actively solicit the input of health professions associations and the education community.

*Implications for nursing education*: Discuss internally at schools of nursing the risks and opportunities of actualizing the five core competencies. Identify the stakeholders in making the change—in most states that would be the institution administration—education and key clinical agencies: chief executive officer (CEO), chief nursing officer (CNO), chief of medicine (COM), deans of the respective health professions colleges, provosts or chancellors, regulatory boards such as the board of nursing or medicine, hospital association, state nursing and medical associations, and board of regents for higher education as well as representatives of community colleges.

3. Building upon previous efforts, accreditation bodies should move forward expeditiously to revise their standards so that programs are required to demonstrate, through process and outcome measures, that they educate students in both academic and continuing education programs in how to deliver patient care using a core set of competencies. In so doing, these bodies should coordinate their efforts.

   *Implications for nursing education*: Educators must work with clinical agencies and state regulatory agencies to form statewide task forces using the model of the workforce task forces to create a consensus document on accreditation changes needed for the new era of health professions education. Next there must be an action plan developed for implementation.

4. All health professions boards should move toward requiring licensed health professionals to demonstrate periodically their ability to deliver patient care, as defined by the five competencies identified by the committee, through direct measures of technical competence, patient assessment, evaluation of patient outcomes, and other evidence-based assessment methods. These boards should simultaneously evaluate the different assessment methods.

   *Implications for nursing education*: Continued competency in practice may become an expectation for teachers, at least in the clinical courses. While this is true at the advanced practice level, it is not at the undergraduate level.

5. Certification bodies should require their certificate holders to maintain their competence throughout their careers by periodically demonstrating their ability to deliver patient care that reflects the five competencies, among other requirements.

   *Implications for nursing education*: Those who teach clinical at any level must demonstrate continued clinical skills and knowledge. Therefore this must be part of the performance evaluation criteria for faculty.

6. Foundations, with support from education and practice organizations, should take the lead in developing and funding regional demonstration learning centers, representing partnerships between practice and education. These centers

should leverage existing innovative organizations and be state-of-the-art training centers focused on teaching and assessing the five core competencies.

*Implications for nursing education*: Create interdisciplinary clinical advisory groups composed of educational institutions (multiple colleges and nursing education systems) and multiple healthcare delivery systems, including state or local health departments, to determine how to develop and implement these learning centers. Key to this implementation is to bring funding agencies into the discussion early to create a cooperative agreement for funding.

7. Through Medicare demonstration projects, the Centers for Medicare and Medicaid Services (CMS) should take the lead in funding experiments to create incentives for health professionals to integrate interdisciplinary approaches into educational or practice settings, with the goal of providing a training ground for students and clinicians that incorporates the five core competencies.

   *Implications for nursing education*: Develop proposals for demonstration projects to examine outcomes of this model. These outcomes would include cost effectiveness, barriers to integration of interdisciplinary models, gaps in knowledge regarding the creation and implementation of these centers, and patient outcomes—morbidity and mortality, safety, and satisfaction.

8. The Agency for Healthcare Research and Quality (AHRQ) and private foundations should support ongoing research projects addressing the five core competencies and their association with individual and population health, as well as research into the link between the competencies and evidence-based education. Such projects should involve researchers across two or more disciplines.

   *Implication for nursing education*: Recognize that health policy is an essential tool for nurses at any level. Use this skill by attending open forums held by AHRQ to voice the new funding needs. Respond to interdisciplinary Requests for Proposals (RFPs) from AHRQ leveraging partnerships with other colleges or healthcare institutions.

9. AHRQ should work with a representative group of healthcare leaders to develop measures reflecting the core set of competencies, set national goals for improvement, and issue a report to the public evaluating progress toward these goals. AHRQ should issue the first report, focused on clinical educational institutions, in 2005 and produce annual reports thereafter.

   *Implication for nursing education*: Involve nursing at the grassroots level to follow the national discussion, determine stakeholders in the state or region, and collectively make a strong voice to AHRQ through the open forums and meetings with key representatives of the agency to shape the agenda for the future.

10. Beginning in 2004, a biennial interdisciplinary summit should be held involving healthcare leaders in education, oversight processes, practice, and other areas. This summit should focus on both reviewing progress against explicit targets and setting goals for the next phase with regard to the five competencies and other areas necessary to prepare professionals for the twenty-first-century health system.

    *Implication for nursing education*: Use key representatives to lobby the nursing and healthcare organizations as well as educational and regulatory bodies to develop state or regional summits to gain an understanding of the needs at these levels. Then take these recommendations to the national level through state medical, nursing, pharmacy, and allied health, and hospital associations so that national summits can be held. The caveat is that this cannot be a ten-year process.

*Source*: Institute of Medicine. (2003). *Health professions education. A bridge to quality*. Washington, DC: The National Academies Press. Reprinted with permission.

# *Appendix J*
# *The IOM Reports: Critical Curricular Content*

The following information from the IOM reports can serve as a guide for critical curricular content to consider when curricula are reviewed and revised.

## *Quality Matrix Dimensions*

*Consumer Perspectives on Healthcare Needs:* Staying healthy, getting better, living with illness or disability, coping with end of life

*Components of Healthcare Quality:* safety, effectiveness, patient centeredness, timeliness

## *Six Improvement Aims*

Health care should be:

(1) Safe
(2) Effective
(3) Patient-centered
(4) Timely
(5) Efficient
(6) Equitable

## *Ten Rules*

(1) Care is based on continuous healing relationships.
(2) Care is customized according to patient needs and values.
(3) Patient is the source of control.
(4) Knowledge is shared and information flows freely.
(5) Decision-making is evidence-based.
(6) Safety is a system property.
(7) Transparency is necessary.

(8) Needs are anticipated.
(9) Waste is continuously decreased.
(10) Cooperation among clinicians is a priority.

See Appendix L, which applies 10 rules to core competencies.

## Six Major Direct-Care Concerns for Nurses

(1) Monitoring patient status or surveillance
(2) Physiological therapy (the most visible intervention that nurses perform)
(3) Helping patients compensate for loss of functioning
(4) Providing emotional support
(5) Education for patients and families
(6) Integration and coordination of care (both related to interdisciplinary teams)

## Priority Areas of Care

- Care coordination (crosses all areas)
- Self-management/health literacy (crosses all areas)
- Asthma: appropriate treatment for persons with mild-to-moderate persistent asthma (related to chronic conditions; children and adolescents)
- Cancer screening that is evidence-based: focus on colorectal and cervical cancer (related to preventive care)
- Children with special healthcare needs at increased risk for chronic physical, developmental, behavioral condition (related to children and adolescents; chronic conditions)
- Diabetes: appropriate management of early disease (related to children and adolescents; chronic conditions)
- End of life with advanced organ system failure: focus on congestive heart failure and chronic obstructive pulmonary disease (related to end of life; chronic conditions; inpatient surgical care)
- Frailty associated with old age: preventing falls and pressure ulcers, maximizing function, and developing advanced care plans (related to end of life; chronic conditions)
- Hypertension: appropriate treatment of early disease (related to preventive care; chronic conditions)
- Immunization: children and adult (related to preventive care; children and adolescents)
- Ischemic heart disease: prevention, reduction of recurring events, and optimization of functional capacity (related preventive care; chronic conditions; inpatient and surgical care)

- Major depression: screening and treatment (related to preventive care screening; behavioral health; children and adolescents)
- Medical management: preventing medication errors and overuse of antibiotics (related to end of life; children and adolescents; chronic conditions; inpatient and surgical care)
- Nosocomial infections: prevention and surveillance (related to end of life; inpatient and surgical care)
- Pain control in advanced cancer (related to end of life; chronic conditions; inpatient and surgical care)
- Pregnancy and childbirth: appropriate prenatal and intrapartum care (related to preventive care; inpatient and surgical care)
- Severe and persistent mental illness: treatment in the public sector (related to behavioral health; chronic conditions; inpatient and surgical care)
- Stroke: early treatment in the public sector (related to chronic conditions; inpatient and surgical care)
- Tobacco dependence: treatment in adults (related to preventive care; behavioral health; chronic conditions)
- Obesity (emerging area or one that affects a broad range of individuals; we still need more information about the best interventions in this area) (related to preventive care; behavioral health; children and adolescents; chronic conditions)

## *Health Professions Core Competencies*

- Provide patient-centered care
- Work in interdisciplinary teams
- Employ evidence-based practice
- Apply quality improvement
- Utilize informatics

# Appendix K

# *Nursing Against* Whose *Odds?* *Commentary on Gordon (2005) as an Example of Teaching to the IOM Reports*

Carole Kenner, DNS, RNC, FAAN,
Dean and Professor, University of Oklahoma College of Nursing

Anita Finkelman, MSN, RN,
Adjunct Faculty, University of Oklahoma College of Nursing

Francene Weatherby, PhD, RNC,
Coordinator, Special Projects, University of Oklahoma College of Nursing

Lisa English Long MSN, RN,
Clinical Nurse Specialist, Cincinnati Children's Hospital Medical Center

Betty R. Kupperschmidt, EdD, RN, CNAA, BC,
Associate Professor, University of Oklahoma College of Nursing, Tulsa

## *Introduction*

Author and journalist Suzanne Gordon has once again taken up the cause of nursing as a profession in her latest book, *Nursing Against the Odds* (2005). This thought–provoking, depressing book portrays the many challenges of nursing today. It uses true accounts from nursing leaders in service and education as well as nurses in the trenches. It tackles everything from victimization and violence, the use of submissive and permissive language, and lack of media savvy to tell the story of health care from a nursing perspective regarding the need for more union representation to avoid the pitfalls of modern day nursing. Whether they agree with the book or not, most nurses can relate to the stories. Gordon touches on crucial issues that deserve professional dialogues with colleagues and students. To that end, representatives from practice and academic settings have accepted the challenge to respond and to highlight the issues from these two arenas. This is a summary of their responses to two questions: *What is your initial reaction to the book?* and *What do you recommend for nursing as a profession?*

This is not meant to be a critical analysis of each of Ms. Gordon's points but rather an example of a discourse that can be used in teaching to begin to delve into professional issues. It is meant to serve as a catalyst for online or face-to-face discussions. It can be used as the basis for a response paper or as a starting point for a critical appraisal of the literature. It is not meant to have the answers or to serve as a critical review. It is a stimulus to get students, faculty, and practitioners talking.

## *What Is Your Initial Reaction to the Book?*

Gordon makes excellent points—many not flattering about nursing, but generally objective comments based on real nursing experiences. Maybe it takes a non-nurse to look into our most difficult professional issues, though Gordon is certainly no stranger to nursing considering her previous publications such as *From Silence to Voice* (Buresh, Gordon, & Jeans, 2003). It is sad that it takes someone outside of nursing to recognize these issues. Nursing education, shortages, relationships with physicians and non-nurse colleagues, Magnet status, and image: all confront nurses every day. When they are discussed by a journalist they seem more powerful. Why? Gordon answers this question in chapter after chapter as she describes our inability to speak with a strong, unified voice. The clear threads through her book are that nursing as a profession needs to stand up and come together to solve the image problem, become the driver of the profession, and act as if nurses are true members of the healthcare team with full status. Our comments focus on the areas that Gordon suggests are the most problematic: education, workplace culture, media image, nursing recruitment and retention, and professionalism.

### Education

Critics claim that nursing education and practice are disconnected. Our educational programs do not match employer expectations. Gordon points out, however, that if we developed curricula truly based on reality, then students might have a serious problem with the National Council Licensure Examination (NCLEX), which is linked to past educational and clinical practices more than to today's healthcare system. The consensus within academe has been not to dilute education by introducing the current state of health care, but instead to hold to high academic standards that may or may not relate to practice. This may sound like a laudable goal, but if nursing schools don't prepare them for the realities of practice, even the highest achieving students may be disillusioned and quit the profession during their first year of employment. Most of us have seen this happen.

Gordon cites the confusion over nursing diagnoses and language. In her view, this language is an inaccurate representation of what nursing contributes to health care. It does not correspond to the language of reimbursement, electronic medical records, charts, and other information systems—physician order entry systems for example. The push for a unified language is global, with the International Council of Nurses (ICN) leading the charge. Many physicians readily admit that they no longer bother to read nursing documentation; they cannot understand it, and feel that nurses are not on the same page as them. Many within our own profession do not understand the language, and some only refer to it because of NCLEX. Some experts agree that the expansion of information mandates a universal systems language, and yet many of these systems do not reflect nursing terminology. So the question becomes if we do not clearly understand what we mean, how can we explain it to others, and if it is not included in information systems, how will nursing care be recorded in the future? This language has value for nursing, to distinguish it from other disciplines, yet it may also extinguish us as a profession. According to Gordon, if nursing students are not taught this language they will struggle with NCLEX. So again we see a disconnect between education and practice.

Students are taught the chain of command for advocating for patients and their families. They are also taught that ultimately nurses cannot diagnose and must defer to physicians. Gordon suggests that what we teach students is a submissive and permissive mentality that instills feelings of powerlessness and victimization, undermining interprofessional teamwork.

In efforts to move away from the medical model and disease orientation, nursing has distanced itself from spheres of influence. Nurses need to learn to communicate with other disciplines and appreciate their unique perspectives, but vague nursing language often obstructs interprofessional work. Nurses need to understand financial models of health care, for example, which is not a strength of many undergraduate nursing programs. Gordon illustrates these problems with her revealing stories of nurses socialized into a lesser status when they have to ask permission to tell a patient something. While they work up the chain of command to get a physician order, another patient may become a failure-to-rescue statistic. This is a disturbing picture of the future of nursing. Who loses? The patient.

Many of the issues raised in this book are really about healthcare safety. In the clinical setting the focus is on safety, and the Institute of Medicine (IOM, 2000, 2004) discusses safety as a key area. In the educational setting, faculty evaluate students on their ability to function safely. Safe practice at any level involves clear communication with patients, families, and all professionals; the nurse's ability to think critically; application of learned knowledge and skills; use of evidence to support practice; and the wisdom to expect the unexpected. This is an important goal, yet we continue to struggle to provide educational experiences that will lead students to the important practice competencies.

### Workplace Culture

This book is deeply disturbing because most nurses can relate to the stories Gordon tells. The themes of victimization, powerlessness, inability to accomplish things in the workplace, and workplace violence are all familiar. It is sad that with all the emphasis on evidence-based practice and Magnet status, and even with evidence of the need for a positive workplace environment, that we are not able to solve these problems in a majority of settings. Gordon's diagnosis—disputes between doctors and nurses are political rather than moral or clinical—has a distinct ring of truth. Her emphatic indictment of embracing *caring* as our moral imperative, the very essence of nursing, also resonated with the reviewers. Several authors, including Porter O'Grady, challenged us some time ago to reconsider that mantra, noting that there is no market for caring per se. To say that doctors cure and nurses care negates the curative aspects of nursing.

Gordon left out two very important issues in her indictment of acute care nursing: the general societal milieu in which nursing care is provided, and the changing nature of patients who come from that culture. She could have cited ample statistics to demonstrate that America is anything but a "kinder, gentler" society. Today there is a general coarsening of interactions among people, which nurses see every day as they work with patients. Patients are understandably under stress: concerned and angry at the amount of their own money they must pay for health care, and dissatisfied with the rotating door aspect of health care. Nurses receive the brunt of these emotions as patients show them not respect but verbal and physical abuse. There is also documentation that nurses do not treat other nurses with respect, although treating each person with respect is the first provision of the ANA Code of Ethics. At the 2006 American Nurses Association House of Delegates, the National Student Nurses president delivered a position statement on horizontal violence. This type of violence is often viewed as "eating our young" or "eating each other." This is a powerful message from our future nurses to those of us already in the profession to reframe our behaviors and critically examine our actions as they relate to our current and future colleagues.

### Media and Nursing Recruitment and Retention

The importance of the media is a theme continued from Gordon's earlier book, *From Silence to Voice* (Buresh, Gordon, & Jeans, 2003). When reporters call schools of nursing or healthcare institutions they are often turned down, sometimes justifiably, but many deserve a courteous response. Gordon suggests that nurses are afraid of reprisals, but often faculty who have no reason for concern will not talk either. When nurses do not appear in the media to describe the role of nursing, this impairs recruitment of future nurses. Again we let someone else speak for us or about us.

We do not articulate what nursing *is* versus what nurses *do*. We still teach students tasks rather than competencies. The thinking, creative student is often penalized and pushed back into the rigid structure that we as faculty present as essential to get through an assignment. Yet in a time of scarce resources, we need critical thinking nurses who can make judgment calls in a highly complex care delivery system. These two positions are diametrically opposed. What employers want, most educators are not prepared to deliver.

Another obstacle to recruitment is the lack of consistent educational pathways to nursing. Some teens do not understand how nurses with only a two-year degree can be respected. Gordon contends that we cannot tackle this issue because we are fragmented. Professional organizations fight among themselves in public when they should debate the issues behind closed doors, reach a consensus, and present a common stance in public. She argues that allied health, pharmacy, and medicine have addressed educational needs and standards far better because they unite when it counts and act as one at a national level. The nursing shortage gives Gordon's refrain of retention and recruitment particular meaning. Until conditions change in hospitals, we in nursing education can produce all the nurses in the world, but new graduates will find the workplace intolerable. Just months after graduation it is not uncommon to hear that nurses are mean to novices, and that novices fear they will make a fatal mistake because there are too many patients and too few nurses. Rather than endure such stress, these new nurses leave not just the institution but the profession. More reasonable workloads, "No Lift" policies, predictable schedules, shared governance, improved nurse–doctor relations, and better pay will go a long way to increase retention and improve nursing's public relations, as Gordon suggests. So in the end we find educators producing graduates without the competencies they need to practice, while healthcare organizations have yet to reform a workplace culture that denies success to novice nurses.

### Professionalism: Dress for Respect

The way we view ourselves, as evidenced by our dress, affects the profession's ability to recruit and retain nurses, our public relations, and our own view of professionalism. Today no common uniform distinguishes the nurse; we have no wish to return to caps and capes and all the rest, but have we gone too far? With everyone in scrubs, most patients cannot tell a nurse from a housekeeper. Furthermore, Gordon suggests that casual dress may induce a casual attitude toward patients and other professionals. Educators generally set standards of appearance for students, such as a clean uniform, no visible tattoos, no facial jewelry, and lab coats in the hospital when not wearing uniforms for clinical experiences. But when they enter the clinical setting, students are confused by staff who do not follow the same standards. The high expectations in the academic setting should continue in the clinical setting, but this does not seem to occur, for as soon as students graduate they follow the dress standards of their new culture. Dress does indicate pride in oneself and influences the respect given a person. It is noteworthy that nursing lost some of its professionalism as dress changed from a professional uniform to scrubs.

## *What Recommendations Do You Have for Nursing as a Profession?*

As a profession we are heading down one path and then there is the other more reality-based path, and they will not meet. The nursing shortage looms, but clearly the shortage is more than people needed to fill slots. Recruitment and retention are major failures. We ourselves are to blame for much of this. We created an Advanced Practice

Nurse (APN) position—"the nurse to be"—and probably lost a lot of nurses who could have been providing direct bedside nursing care today.

We have dutifully chanted "community care," and yet we have sicker and sicker patients in acute care as well as in the community or home. Home care agencies are not looking for nurses steeped in the community, they need nurses with excellent acute care skills. We have told students that the community is where care is delivered, but there are few openings. Many community jobs, such as home care, hospice, and ambulatory care, require acute care experience. Many nurse educators do not even consider these community settings—they are looking for population-based experience, which is truly hard to find. We have not approached education about community care effectively. We scramble for clinical experiences, doing a few days here and there. Community experiences may include conducting wellness screenings, then spending a few days in a school where the nursing students sit around with little to do unless by great good luck a school nurse has created an innovative program, then participating in clinic visits where the registered nurses is the traffic manager, and then some home care experience. Home care can be one the best community experiences, and yet it is not used consistently.

As we fumble to figure out roles and best education experiences, healthcare delivery goes on. Nurses provide care, and hopefully patients improve, though recent data indicates that health care has a serious error rate (IOM, 2000).

What is the message from this book? Bluntly, RN substitutes will take our places if we do not get off the dime and face these problems. Like Gordon, many of us would feel safer if we could take an RN to the hospital with us. Yet what are we as educators and practicing nurses doing to change that? Students have a tough time gaining clinical experience because we hold to the traditional ways of teaching labs and rotating through numerous healthcare settings, when the only thing being learned in the first several weeks is not nursing care but where the bathrooms are, how to chart, and the code for the medication system. Clinical days with long gaps between them do not allow students to experience caregiving over an extended period; rather, students often see a rapid turnover of patients who are gone when they return.

On the practice side we are often unwilling to give up tasks that someone else could do, tasks that do not involve nursing assessment and judgment. The public is beginning to understand that nurses are there 24/7 and are the glue that holds health care together. They see the enormous responsibility we have. Why don't we see the power?

We need to break out of our silos, support our practice with evidence, and collaborate with all team members to promote the best outcomes for our patients and families. We tend to work *alongside* all other services or disciplines as opposed to working *with* them. We may blame it on them (usually the physicians) but perhaps we need to reach across the aisle and invite them to work with us. This would promote interdisciplinary or interprofessional work and improve outcomes. It would take effort on several fronts. For example, in one healthcare organization the physician group has a badge reader outside each conference room; presently the badge reader only approves physician badges, so nurses are locked out. The clinical director has had no luck in changing this. The issues of victimization, leveling, and professionalism discussed in the book feel very personal. We as nurses need to learn how to deal with situations like this and how to use positive confrontation to maneuver through the system and reach successful outcomes.

Collaboration is critical. To improve patient outcomes, we need to bring healthcare professionals together to solve problems and arrive at solutions; that should begin on the first day of orientation. Bedside nurses should always be involved in patient rounds, during which they should have an active part in decision-making. We need to make every effort to increase opportunities to collaborate within our profession and interprofessionally rather than wait for opportunities to come to us. We need leadership.

Nurses (individually and as a profession) have done a very ineffective job of documenting the difference that nurses make to acute care, both in treatment of patients and in cost control. Although there is a national emphasis on evidence-based practice (EBP), nurses still say, "But everybody knows . . ." We have to replace that rhetoric with "The evidence shows . . . " Then maybe we can silence "ain't it awful" books like this one. We must also find a way to ensure that baccalaureate-prepared nurses do not regress to the mean in acute care. Concurrently, we must document the difference that nurses with BSN and graduate degrees make wherever patient care is delivered, but especially in the troubled arena of acute care. We need to immerse nurses in EBP by encouraging nurses to ask the clinical questions, providing education in the EBP process, and establishing a system to support them in leading or participating in an EBP project. If we do this, we can speak the same language as our colleagues in medicine (they are farther along in this process), support our practice, and challenge those who continue to direct us to do it "the way it has always been done."

While these BSN-prepared nurses role-model professional nursing practice, they must not adopt a superior attitude toward their other team members. Appreciate that *we each* have the opportunity to change things if we want to. We don't have to wait for someone else to do it or feel at the mercy of "the administration" to change things. The issue of technical vs. professional is ever present. Gordon observes that certain subject matter is covered for some programs and not for others, and then asks why all RN programs don't include the same content if they provide the same care. We know this question of consistency has never been resolved by having all of us take the same NCLEX. The other part of this argument is that of those master's degree graduates we produce, many are now being recruited by nontraditional, often better paying opportunities in corporations, research and development companies, and legal nurse consulting firms, and away from direct care and education. Whose fault is this?

To address some of these education and practice issues, the educator must consider the need to:

- Instill respect for individuals. Show students they are valued and respected and that this is something they should expect.

- Address students with language fitting to our profession, and present a professional appearance.
- Have faculty discuss selected chapters from the book to increase faculty awareness of how these issues affect interactions with students.
- Make interactions with bedside nursing experts more visible.
- Increase interdisciplinary and interprofessional learning interactions with the medical school and other allied health professions.
- Increase media coverage of nursing, including nursing students and nursing education.

Books like this impede collaboration between acute care nursing (as embodied by the American Organization of Nurse Executives) and the professional nursing camp (predominantly the American Nurses Association). That can be a decided detriment to the profession. Yet this book should spark dialogue among various nursing groups. Physician–nurse turf disputes need to be resolved. If we do not accomplish this, we will never move forward as a profession. Certainly, much needs to change on the medical end, but we have to take responsibility for ourselves. Nursing faculty need to stop disparaging physicians in the classroom and instead foster collaboration and confrontation of issues, not people, in order to enhance communication. We all care about the patient, yet this is difficult to recognize in the classroom or in the clinical setting on some days, especially when we teach and learn in silos. Gordon comments on how we tend to frame things from a moral stance and avoiding talking about clinical issues, strategies, and so on. We have a long history of "put downs": technical nurses vs. professional nurses, APN nurses vs. clinical specialists, APN vs. direct care and acute care nurses. The recent IOM reports, particularly *Health Professions Education* (IOM, 2003), identify five core competencies, one of which is teamwork. We cannot teach teamwork as we have. We need to include teamwork in every course we teach and in clinical experiences. From day one of any health profession education, we need to "cross the street" to the college of medicine or any other health profession and say, "We are here to figure out how we can focus on teamwork and communication across disciplines."

It can be done, but it will take added effort for some nurse educators to move away from the stance that physicians are the bad guys. We can say teamwork is the responsibility of the healthcare organization, but this is not so; their responsibility is to support teamwork in the healthcare setting. Healthcare providers should come to the work setting with the competencies necessary to work on a team to provide physical care to patients while others often do not.

We have caught ourselves in another vise in nursing education. Academia wants faculty to have PhDs. That would be nice, but it is not happening. The tenure track causes major problems in nursing education. Why? The system is a class system. Those without a PhD who do most of the teaching are considered to be the workers. Some clinical faculty say, "We are the slaves. Tenured and tenure-track faculty sit in their offices and pretend to do research." Now, do we want faculty who have not been in the healthcare setting for a long time to teach?

The severe shortage of faculty will continue. However, we have not seriously considered whether we are effectively using the faculty we have. This would not totally solve the shortage, but it could make a difference.

We must respect members of other professions and those within our own profession. Faculty must respect each other. Too often it is implied that tenured and tenure-track faculty are better than clinical faculty, when in reality each has strengths and weaknesses. Working together for the good of the profession and the students' education, we will set students an example they can carry into their professional careers.

This book should stimulate the profession to discuss these issues and meet them squarely with action plans. Partnerships between clinical and educational areas are critical ways to begin this dialogue. One wonders whether we are a genuine practice discipline when many faculty are no longer in touch with clinical settings. We need to remember the 1970s and the call for one strong voice for nursing. There is a place for specialty organizations, but when difficult issues arise we need to keep our fights behind closed doors, and in public present a united front. Of course, this means that we need a mechanism for speedy consensus building among constituencies. We need to learn how to give in on small points and quickly identify the hills to die for. We do not play well together, and this hurts us tremendously in the bigger political arena. We cannot blame all this on physicians and healthcare organizations because they can only take away as much power as we are willing to give up. We need to prepare the next generation of nurses for the real world and not the ivory tower version. We need to teach them about finances and politics and why they need to care. We need to teach them why it is important to belong to a professional organization, because today the majority do not, and this requires that practicing nurses and educators act as role models by joining and participating, and then draw in students and new graduates.

What will this take? The following professional strategies are a start:

- *Establish and promote an atmosphere* where nurses can *care*, *think critically*, ask the *clinical questions*, and initiate *change* to improve the outcomes for their patients and themselves.
- *Work together as nurses and with allies.* This is a complex problem that requires multiple strategies.
- *Remember our roots.* Showcase the traditional skills, knowledge, and expertise of the bedside nurse.
- *Emphasize the knowledge of nursing.* Since this aspect of nursing has been downplayed, as Gordon notes, it will need greater stress to gain ground. But care should be taken not to denigrate the caring aspects of nursing. The human aspect, the caring portion of a nursing career, is what draws many into the profession. It is what patients say they appreciate about nursing, and what

they see lacking in the care they receive from most doctors. So make sure caring is included—skilled, informed caring. Given a choice of expert knowledge and skill or a compassionate, caring attitude, any rationale person would choose the expert knowledge and skill. But why should any patient have to choose just one? The expert nurse should provide a blend of both.

## *Conclusion*

According to Gordon, it will take all of us working together to raise nursing from the slump we are in to a more promising future. We need to encourage junior faculty to share their success stories with colleagues and to work cooperatively with other faculty. We must challenge our colleagues to embrace change, to revise curricula to meet changing expectations, to learn about pilot projects such as the Clinical Nurse Leader (CNL), and to remain current in the nursing literature.

The book as a whole would make an excellent text for a health policy course—all of the course on critical health policy issues or a professional issues forum. In these two areas students and faculty could debate the issues and explore other sources to confirm or refute their positions. The answers to these hard questions begin with education. Every issue we face stems from the education nurses receive, and not just the curriculum. The interactions and role modeling that faculty provide, the clinical experiences, strategies for success, critical thinking, collaboration, conflict resolution, and professionalism—all are necessary parts of a nurse's education.

More than focusing on the problems, this book should challenge us to appreciate that we have the power (individually and collectively) to change the future of nursing. Are we up to the challenge?

## *References*

Buresh, B., Gordon, S., & Jeans, M. (2003). *From silence to voice.* Ithaca, NY: Cornell University Press.

Gordon, S. (2005). *Nursing against the odds.* Ithaca, NY: Cornell University Press.

Institute of Medicine (IOM). (2000). *To err is human.* Washington, DC: National Academies Press.

Institute of Medicine (IOM). (2003). *Health professions education.* Washington, DC: National Academies Press.

Institute of Medicine (IOM). (2004). *Keeping patients safe.* Washington, DC: National Academies Press.

# Appendix L
## Clinical Prevention and Population Health: Curricular Framework for Health Professions

- Core Component: Evidence Base of Practice
  - Epidemiology and biostatistics
    Rates of disease, types of data, statistical concepts
  - Methods for evaluating health research literature
    Study designs, quality measures, sampling and statistical power
  - Outcome measurement, including quality and costs
    Measures that include quality of life or utility, measures that include cost, measures of quality of health care
  - Health surveillance
    Vital statistics, disease surveillance, biological, social, economic, geographic, and behavioral risk factors
  - Determinants of health
    Burden of illness, contributors to morbidity and mortality
- Core Component: Clinical Prevention Services, Health Promotion
  - Screening
    Approaches to testing and screening, criteria for successful screening, evidence-based recommendations
  - Counseling
    Approaches to culturally appropriate behavioral change, clinician–patient communication, criteria for successful counseling, evidence-based recommendations
  - Immunizations
    Approaches to vaccination, criteria for successful immunizations, evidence-based recommendations
  - Chemoprevention
    Approaches to chemoprevention, criteria for successful chemoprevention, evidence-based recommendations

- Core Component: Health Systems and Health Policy
  - Organization of clinical and public health systems
    Clinical health services, public health responsibilities, relationship between clinical practice and public health
  - Health services financing
    Clinical services coverage and reimbursement, methods of financing healthcare institutions, methods of financing public health services, other models (international)
  - Health workforce
    Methods of regulation of professions and health care, discipline-specific history, philosophy, roles and responsibilities, racial and ethnic workforce composition including under-represented minorities, relations of discipline to other healthcare professionals, legal and ethical responsibilities of healthcare professionals
  - Health policy process
    Process of health policy-making, methods of participation in the policy process, impact of policies on health care and health outcomes including impacts on vulnerable populations
- Core Component: Community Aspects of Practice
  - Communicating and sharing health information with the public
    Methods of assessing community needs or strengths and options for intervention, media communications, evaluation of health information
  - Environmental health
    Sources, media, and routes of exposure to environmental contaminants, environmental health risk assessment and risk management, environmental disease prevention focusing on susceptible populations
  - Occupational health
    Risks from employment-based exposures, methods for control of occupational exposures, exposure and prevention in healthcare settings
  - Global health issues
    Roles of international organizations, disease and population patterns in other countries, effects of globalization on health
  - Cultural dimensions of practice
    Cultural influences on clinician's delivery of health services, cultural influences on individuals and communities, culturally competent health care
  - Community services
    Methods of facilitating access to and partnerships for health care, evidence-based recommendations for community prevention services, public health preparedness

*Source*: Allan, J., et al. (2004). Clinical Prevention and Population Health: Curriculum Framework for Health Professions. *American Journal of Preventive Medicine, 27*(5), 471–476. Reprinted with permission.

# Index